THE
SECRETS
OF
PAIN RELIEF

THE
SECRETS
OF
PAIN RELIEF

NATURAL REMEDIES THAT WILL END YOUR SUFFERING

DR. LUIS ALIAGA

Translated by Allison Hauptman

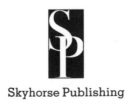

Skyhorse Publishing

First published in Spain by Grupo Océano in 2011.
Original title: VENCER EL DOLOR DE FORMA NATURAL
© Luis Aliaga Font, 2011
© Editorial Océano, S. L., 2012 (Barcelona, Spain)
Ocean Group Milanesat 21-23—08017 Barcelona
Tel: 93 280 20 20—Fax: 93 203 17 91
www.oceano.com

All inquiries should be addressed to Skyhorse Publishing, 307 West 36th Street, 11th Floor, New York, NY 10018.

Skyhorse Publishing books may be purchased in bulk at special discounts for sales promotion, corporate gifts, fund-raising, or educational purposes. Special editions can also be created to specifications. For details, contact the Special Sales Department, Skyhorse Publishing, 307 West 36th Street, 11th Floor, New York, NY 10018 or info@skyhorsepublishing.com.

Skyhorse® and Skyhorse Publishing® are registered trademarks of Skyhorse Publishing, Inc.®, a Delaware corporation.

Visit our website at www.skyhorsepublishing.com.

10 9 8 7 6 5 4 3 2 1

Library of Congress Cataloging-in-Publication Data is available on file.

Cover design by Jane Sheppard
Interior images by iStock

ISBN: 978-1-5107-0552-4
eBook ISBN: 978-1-5107-0557-9

33614057653841

Printed in the United States of America

Contents

Introduction

Pain, in one form or another, has always been a part of human life. Throughout history, mankind has sought solutions to help alleviate all kinds of pain, but we have only achieved partial or temporary relief. In the twenty-first century, experts still consider chronic pain one of the most concerning health problems affecting the population. Many of those who suffer musculoskeletal discomfort are not satisfied with their treatment. Seeing as over half of the population will suffer from arthritis or another rheumatic disease at some point in their life, this is not a very hopeful future.

Chronic pain can affect anyone. Throughout history, we have seen records from kings to painters, musicians to inventors, who have suffered from severe pain. Charles V, Holy Roman Emperor, suffered from severe attacks of gout that left him with a great physical disability; Christopher Columbus who lived for years in intense pain, suffering from strange symptoms, died at age fifty-four; and Sergei Rachmaninov, the last of the Romantic composers, though he suffered such severe pain that he could no longer compose music, discovered that performing on stage helped relieve the discomfort. Freud had migraines, Frida Kahlo was diagnosed with chronic pain, and Renoir had arthritis.

Many of those suffering from chronic pain feel misunderstood when they try to describe their symptoms, whether to their family, friends, or doctors. Often, their pain will be underestimated and left untreated. As a subjective sensation, pain is difficult to demon-strate. Patients are often passed from one specialist to another, only to be prescribed NSAIDS (nonsteroidal anti-inflammatories) to alleviate their chronic pain.

According to studies, it takes an average of two years for a patient to get proper treatment. Suffering from chronic pain for more than six months multiplies the risk of psychosocial impairment and disability, and causes a significant decrease in quality of life.

A study conducted in Spain on a population of five thousand people showed that 29 percent of the study's participants had pain the day before the study, and 43 percent reported having pain the week before the study. The incidence of pain increased with age, reaching 42 percent in people over sixty-five years old claiming that they suffered from pain daily. Professor Paul Langley of the University of Minnesota conducted the study "Pain in Europe" in 2003, which included more than fifty thousand people from various European countries. The study showed that 19 percent of participants suffered from chronic pain. This represents about 75 million people over the age of forty. In Spain, the percentage of people suffering from chronic pain was only recorded to be 12 percent; could this be because of the difference in lifestyle, food, and recreational activity?

In the United States, about 30 percent of the population suf-fers from back pain. About 70 million Americans develop chronic pain annually, with more than 50 million suffering partial or total debilitation ranging from days to months, or in some cases, for life.

In 1900, the average life expectancy was between 31 and 50 years, and as of 2005, it was between 65 and 80. It is estimated that the pop-ulation over the age of 64 will make up 37 percent of the population by 2030, and 60 percent by 2049. This demographic change is being called a "demographic tsunami." The prevalence of diseases related to aging will increase dramatically in the United States and Europe. Pain will need to be treated in order to live a long life.

Pain has a great socioeconomic impact and is among one of the ten diseases that most impact healthcare budgets, as stated by Professor Ceri Philips of the School of Health Sciences at Swansea University (UK). Pain not only affects the patient (through the cost of their treatment, loss of leisure time, deterioration in the quality of life, etc.), but the health system (through examinations, therapies, consultations, etc.), and society in general (lost productivity, stress, etc.).

Back pain is one of the leading causes of absenteeism. In the UK, back pain is responsible for 12.3 billion euros or 22 percent of the total cost of health care.

What can be done to combat this health problem? Most specialists recommend physical exercise (adapted to each patient and supervised by the specialist in rehabilitation) as a tool to help prevent disability related to pain or to restore function.

Research in this area is showing progress. Americans David Julius and Linda Watkins and Israeli Baruch Minke have won the 2012 Prince of Asturias Prize of Scientific and Technical Research for their innovative studies on pain. The jury noted that the winners "have made discoveries that together allow a deeper understanding of cellular and molecular bases of the different sensations, especially pain." The World Association for the Study of Pain and associations on state and local levels provide places where patients can discuss their doubts and concerns. It is also important to mention the proliferation of pain clinics which work toward the aim of finding solutions to different types of pain.

I am honored to run the Teknon Pain Clinic, a multidisciplinary center whose objective is the diagnosis, management, and treatment of chronic pain (from cancer- and non-cancer-related conditions). The Teknon Pain Clinic provides pharmacological or interventional procedures for chronic pain and for rehabilitation. Teams provide a comprehensive evaluation of the patient and create individualized therapy tailored to each patient to help them live their lives without pain.

Through our partnership with the Millennium Pain Center of Chicago, we have become one of the few private teams that have both a basic and clinical research department. We are up to date on all the latest techniques and procedures, scientific research, and cutting-edge treatments for chronic pain.

I have over thirty years of experience in the field of pain research and treatment, and with the collaboration of Cedor Enrich, we have created this book. This project is made possible by Grupo Océano, and with the help of the other experienced members of my team, Drs. Carlos Nebrada, Antonio Ojeda, and María Teresa Vincente, and with the collaboration of journalist Carlota Máñez. We have worked for months to make this abstract and complex subject accessible to readers, through a practical and enjoyable book. Anyone suffering from pain or looking to help a loved one can find answers and guidance in this manual.

To all my team and Carlota Máñez, thank you very much.

Dr. Luis Aliaga
Director of Anesthesiology Services
Clinical Coordinator, Teknon Pain Clinic
(www.teknon.es/clinicadolor/equipo.htm)
Teknon Medical Center, Barcelona
(Associated Millennium Pain Center of Chicago)
(clinicadolor@teknon.es)

Book completed in February 2012
in Pereira Parda (Galdo, Lugo)

A Little Theory

Dr. Antonio Ojeda, Dr. Carlos Nebreda, Dr. Luis Aliaga

Mankind has always experienced pain. All of us at some point in our lives has endured a painful experience.

But what is pain? There are countless definitions. The Spanish Royal Academy describes it as a disturbing and distressing sensation of a body part by internal or external cause. This definition refers both to the physical and emotional aspects of pain. The World Association for the Study of Pain defines it as "an unpleasant sensory and emotional experience associated with actual or potential tissue damage." To better understand this definition, it is necessary to understand the two components that define pain. The first, sensory, refers to the painful feeling; and the second component which is associated with pain suffering.

There are several classifications of the types of pain. The most common way to classify pain is to differentiate between acute pain and chronic pain. The distinction between these two types of pain goes beyond the length of time the pain is experienced, as discussed below.

Acute pain is crucial to our survival because it acts as a biological alarm system that warns us that something is causing harm to our body. It occurs when a harmful stimulus triggers a series of responses to defend our body. These responses include quick reflexes, such as the pulling away of the affected limb, or muscle contraction; and the production of hormones like epinephrine which prepares us to deal with a threat. Acute pain disappears after the root cause is eliminated and should last less than six months.

According to the IASP, chronic pain is pain that lasts for more than six months, while Dr. John J. Bonica defines chronic pain as pain that persists a month after the injury. Acute pain is a symptom of a disease, while chronic pain is the disease itself.

In addition, pain can be classified according to the physio-pathological mechanism that produces nociceptive and neuro-pathic pain. This classification is particularly useful because we know that the treatment of each of these types of pain varies significantly. Nociceptive pain is produced when a stimulus causes damage or injury to internal tissues (somatic pain) or external tissues (visceral pain). It is the result of the activation of a specific system, starting with peripheral receptors and ending with the interpretation of the signal in the brain. Neuropathic pain is when the pain caused by injury or disease is not harmful, but the stimuli feel it as though it is harmful. That is, the body interprets abnormal signals, creating pain specific to certain stimuli.

> When pain becomes chronic, when it loses its protective purpose, it becomes a problem.

HOW DO WE FEEL PAIN?

Acute pain occurs with the activation of the small nerve endings specifically developed to feel the noxious stimuli. These endings are nociceptors, located along the whole body, both in the skin and deeper organs (visceral and musculoskeletal nociceptors).

They can be triggered by mechanical, thermal, or chemical stimuli. Stimuli captured by nociceptors travel through the nerve body to the nerve cell fibers (neuronal soma) located in an anatomical structure (dorsal root ganglion) that is close to the spine. From here they travel through the spinal cord (dorsal horn), where the neurons communicate through chemicals called "neurotransmitters." In the spinal cord, these nerve fibers are arranged in packets called "bundles" (spinothalamic), and target structures in the brain. Among these is the thalamus, which acts as the gateway of information to the cerebral cortex. It can determine whether a stimulus is painful, as well as the pain intensity, and thus the suffering caused by the painful stimulus is perceived. Then the signals travel to the cerebral cortex, which analyzes all the painful information.

It is necessary to point out that the downward path of pain is to regulate the function of the upward transmission of nociceptive impulses (from the periphery to the brain), constituting a sort of filter for different stimuli. The most important transmitters are endogenous opioids, glutamate (an amino acid that acts as a powerful excitatory neurotransmitter), and inhibitory circuits, especially those related to GABA (gamma-Aminobutyric acid), which is the principal cerebral inhibitory neurotransmitter, and glycine (an amino acid that acts as potent inhibitory neurotransmitter).

HOW ARE NOCICEPTORS ACTIVATED?

The presence of tissue injury is necessary for nociceptor activation to produce an inflammatory response with the consequent production of a series of chemical reactions. Serotonin, histamine, prostaglandins and substance P, and neurotransmitters such as acetylcholine, norepinephrine, epinephrine can all cause this reaction. Physical and chemical changes such as changes in pH, temperature changes, or changes in the osmolarity of the medium can also activate nociceptors.

Another feature of these substances is that they are capable of producing a phenomenon known as "sensitization" which is to change the structure of the receptor to be more like these molecules. They also activate phospholipase, an enzyme capable of transforming lipids of cell membranes in arachidonic acid, which is the precursor of a group of chemical mediators known as "prostaglandins" and "thromboxane," many of which also act as nociceptor sensitizers. Cyclooxygenase is the enzyme necessary for this reaction. It is important to know because it is it is targeted by analgesics such as aspirin and ibuprofen.

It is also important to know that the pain threshold is the minimum stimulus it takes to perceive the sensation. For example, most people begin to feel a painful stimulus when the thermal temperature reaches 120 degrees Fahrenheit. Similarly, a mechanical stimulus will begin to feel painful when a certain degree of pressure is applied. Pain tolerance is defined as the maximum level of pain a person is able to endure. This level varies dramatically from person to person and is influenced by emotional factors such as previous experience, personality, and sociocultural influences.

WHERE IS PAIN LOCATED?

The location of pain depends on the type of pain. In the case of surface peripheral nociceptive pain, which is encoded by nociceptors of the skin, mucous membranes and subcutaneous tissue, the pain is usually localized, throbbing or pulsing if the stimulation is brief, or burning if the stimulation is more prolonged. The deep nociceptive pain comes from the excitement of the osteoarticular receptors and is usually more difficult to locate and is characterized by a duller, diffused pain. Alternatively, visceral nociceptive pain, which is what occurs when there is damage to an internal organ, is often vague, fuzzy, difficult to locate, and accompanied by other symptoms such as sweating, nausea or changes in heart rate, and can cause pain in other regions beside the affected one.

This type of pain is present in a different region than the injured area (e.g., shoulder pain during a heart attack). It is believed to be caused when the nerve endings in the affected region cause the same level of pain in the spinal cord, resulting in the central nervous system interpreting the perceived pain coming from two regions.

We must differentiate between this type of pain and pain projection, which occurs when there is a stimulus to a nerve in a more central point with respect to the projector body. That is, the injury to the central location can be felt in the periphery of the nerve. This happens in the sciatic nerve, in which pain in the lower extremities is caused by compression of a nerve at the base of the spine.

HOW COMMON IS PAIN?

Pain is one of the main reasons for medical consultation. Different studies discuss a wide prevalence of pain, found among 19 percent to 81 percent of patients. This broad range is associated with major methodological differences between the various scientific studies, the different definitions used, the use of various measurement scales and the study of different types of patients.

Various reports done on the study of chronic pain note a prevalence of chronic pain in between 17 percent and 40 percent of the population. Despite the differences between each case observed, it is certain that chronic pain is a serious problem in today's society, causing not only an economic burden due to disability, but also affecting the patient's interpersonal relationships and environment, worsening their health and causing further suffering. This scourge is far from being solved and remains undervalued and undertreated.

IS PAIN SUBJECTIVE?

The perception of pain is complex and involves not just biological responses that occur after contact with a harmful stimulus, but also emotional factors that vary from person to person. These factors include previous experience, personality, and sociocultural factors. Therefore pain is always subjective and varies according to each person and each type of pain.

There are clinical differences in how men and women perceive pain. Women are, for example, at a higher risk of developing certain types of painful syndromes such as fibromyalgia and chronic migraines, they are more sensitive to induced pain, and they consult doctors more often. This difference comes from previous experiences, also with hormonal factors playing a major role. Because of these subjective differences, perception of pain also varies between different races and people of different ages.

We know that children tend to perceive painful stimuli with greater intensity than adults. Children, depending on age, have little to no experience with pain, and are suffering this sort of pain for the first time. Regardless of the degree of damaged tissue, this can be perceived as the greatest pain suffered thus far in their lives. On the other hand, with regard to nociceptive receptors, these differences can be explained by the immaturity of the nervous system, causing the child to be unable to discriminate painless stimuli from painful stimuli. "Neuroplasticity" describes the ability of neurons to adapt to different situations, and when it comes to children, their nociceptive system has a lot of plasticity. Therefore they feel painless or slightly painful stimuli, and experience pain or perceived injury.

IS PAIN GENETIC?

A study was published at the beginning of 2005 in the medical journal of Human Molecular Genetics coordinated by Dr. L. Davidenko at the University of North Carolina in the United States in which a gene whose different haplotypes influence the sensitivity and risk of developing a painful chronic illness in the temporomandibular joint. The gene studied was the gene responsible for coding the enzyme catecholamine-O-methyltransferase (an enzyme involved in the synthesis of epinephrine, norepinephrine and dopamine), which are important neurotransmitters.

Children perceive painful stimuli that evokes tissue damage with more intensity.

This study shows that in the near future, we may be able to determine which individuals are at an increased risk of developing chronic pain, and this may help develop individualized therapeutic interventions from the pharmocogenetic field to prevent and treat this disease. This discovery also opens the door to genetic research about whether pain is isolated in certain genes linked to other chronic pain conditions.

PAIN THROUGHOUT HISTORY

Pain is linked inseparably to being human, creating a complex historical journey of this phenomenon. To illustrate this statement, we can look to the Old Testament, Genesis, wherein the third chapter reads "give birth to your children in pain." Or refer to the first of the four noble truths that are the essence of Buddhist doctrine, in which it is stated that suffering and pain are universal, and no one can be free of this from birth to death.

For primitive man, only pain caused by an external occurrence had a clear explanation. Pain caused by an illness was difficult to understand, and they attributed this to a punishment from the gods or possession by spirits or demons in the body. They treated external pain with plants, animal blood, heating or cooling, with magical rites, and blocking holes in the body where spirits and demons could enter.

In ancient civilizations—such as the Assyrians, Babylonians, Egyptians and Hebrews—pain had a religious connotation, and was considered an intoxication by evil spirits, or a punishment from their gods. Ancient Chinese theories called pain a loss of balance between yin and yang within the patient's heart. In 2600 BC, Huang Ti produced anesthesia from medicinal plants, such as hashish, and used acupuncture to help with pain.

In India, it was believed that pain was caused by the frustration of desires and was located in the soul. They were one of the first cultures to emphasize the importance of the psychological component of pain.

There are records dating back to ancient Mesopotamia about the treatment of pain. Since 4000 BC, the Sumerians used the "plant of joy," referring to the poppy. This is the first historical reference of the use of opium. In Sumerian tablets found in Nippur (2250 BC), they discuss the use of medicinal plants for the treatment of pain. Similarly, the Ebers Papyrus (1550 BC), the most important medical document from ancient Mesopotamia which is preserved today, describes in detail the use of opium for headaches brought upon the sufferer by the god Ra.

There is also archeological evidence of the consumption of opium by the ancient Greeks during the Trojan War (1200 BC). The Greek sages theorized about what causes pain, and where it comes from. The theory put forth by Aristotle says that pain travels through the skin via the bloodstream to the heart, and he argued that pain was a disturbance of the heart's temperature in turn determined by the brain. This theory was maintained for more than twenty-three centuries.

Hippocrates (460–377 BC), father of medicine and the greatest doctor in ancient Greece, considered pain to be a disturbance of balance in the heart, and proposed the use of a *spongia somnifera*—a sea sponge soaked in opium, henbane, and mandrake—and also described the use of white willow bark (which contains precursors to aspirin) for the treatment of pain related to childbirth.

In the Greek era, there are descriptions of the use of fish (such as eels), capable of delivering electric shocks for the treatment of nerve pain. This is the beginning of using electrical stimulation for the treatment of pain.

In ancient Rome, Galen (130–200 BC) wrote an amazing description of the nervous system and its direct relation to cerebral pain.

Avicenna, the great Persian doctor of the eleventh century, indicated that pain receptors are located in the brain in the anterior ventricle. He classified many different painkillers, with opium being the strongest, and cold water and ice ranking the least potent. He used opium frequently. It is believed that he died in the year 1037 of an overdose.

On the other side of the world in 400–700 BC, we have the pre-Columbian American civilizations. The Incas had been using coca leaves on wounds to help with the pain, which is considered the first local anesthetic. The Mayans used Jimson weed (a plant that contains scopolamine and atropine) as a painkiller during childbirth. In their society, they conflated pain with death.

In the Renaissance, Leonardo da Vinci created an anatomical drawing of the nerves in the human body and their relation to pain, confirming the theories of Galen. Descartes, in his 1664 book *L'Homme*, put forth the idea that pain travels through thin strands, supporting the theories of Galen and discrediting Aristotle.

With the rise of science (especially in anatomy, physics, and chemistry) in the eighteenth century, the treatment of pain was totally empirical and scientific, leading to modern anesthesia and pharmacological painkillers.

At this point, we should note that the history of pain treatment and the history of modern anesthesia go hand-in-hand. This can be observed in the different definitions of the specialties. For example, the American Society of Anesthesiology (ASA), defines the practice of medicine dedicated to the relief of pain and total patient care, before, during, and after surgery.

The advance of modern chemistry and understanding of the properties of gases that treat pain in turn encouraged the development of anesthesia. However, in the eighteenth century, nitrous oxide was considered a deadly gas. Nonetheless, in 1796, a pharmacist's apprentice and surgical assistant, Humphry Davy, inhaled this gas and had a pleasant experience. He explained that this gas was capable of relieving pain, and it was then used at parties socially, losing credibility in the scientific world.

It was not until March 30, 1842 when a rural doctor and dentist in Georgia, Crawford Williamson Long, described the administration of ether to a friend while extracting a neck tumor without causing pain. It was rumored in various circles in the city that Dr. Long put his patients' lives in danger, and his discovery was not well received. His contemporary, Horace Wells, began to use nitrous oxide as an anesthetic. He used this gas in public demonstrations and realized that the people on whom he was using it experienced less pain, so he decided to see these effects for himself. December 11, 1844, after inhaling the gas, his assistant John Riggs pulled a tooth without Wells feeling any pain. Dr. Wells prepared a public exhibition that was a failure, and he lost all credibility. On October 16, 1846 in Massachusetts, Dr. Morton, a student of Dr. Wells, made the first successful public demonstration of the use of gas (in this case, ether), as an anesthetic and painkiller. This is considered the first successful use of general anesthesia in history.

Thomas Morton was recognized by the scientific community at the time. Years later, March 30th was named Doctor's Day, to celebrate the original discovery by Crawford Williamson Long.

At the beginning of the nineteenth century, Sertürner (1783–1841) managed to isolate the substance opium. When he administrated this to animals, it made them sleep; he named it "morphine" after Morpheus, the god of sleep.

In 1859, Albert Nieman was able to isolate cocaine from the leaves of the coca plant. This substance began to be used in a significant manner as a local anesthetic. In 1885, Leonard Corning created an epidural anesthetic by injecting a solution of cocaine crystals into the patient's back. In 1898, Dr. Augusto Bier developed the concept of administering a cocaine anesthetic in the spine. And in 1899, Felix Hofmann, a chemist who worked for Bayer, isolated acetylsalicylic acid (aspirin). Later, in 1904, the first local anesthesic was produced: novocaine. In 1921, a Spanish army surgeon, Fidel Pagés, proposed the use of lumbar epidural blocks and named it "metameric anesthesia".

Dr. John J. Bonica was one of the first to highlight the possibility that pain can be treated from a multidisciplinary point of view. This idea was crucial. In 1953, he wrote a textbook exclusively dedicated to pain management, and in 1960, he created the first multidisciplinary pain clinic in Seattle, which has served as a model for pain clinics around the world.

Another important discovery came in 1965, when Drs. Patrick D. Wall and Ronald Melzack described the gate control theory, recognizing the nervous system as a modulator of sensory information. They described the pain pathways and established the existence of the central and peripheral nervous system.

Presently, the field of pain research is of great scientific importance, making progress in discoveries such as the role of NMDA receptors (N-methyl D-aspartate), and in 1991, the central sensitization, or the identification of genes predisposed to the development of various chronic pain conditions.

How and When Does Pain Become Chronic?

Dr. Antonio Ojeda, Dr. Luis Aliaga

As we have seen, acute pain is necessary for our survival. It is a protective mechanism that alerts us to dangerous situations, lets us develop reflexes, and helps us create strategies to avoid harmful stimuli. In a nutshell, acute pain is a defense mechanism that advises us and prepares us to face danger.

But how and when does pain, which has such a useful function in dangerous situations, stop being helpful and become a real problem?

To discuss this subject, we need to begin with the definition of chronic pain. The most common definition indicates that pain becomes chronic after six months. Another accepted definition is that chronic pain is pain that continues after the cause is absent, and characteristically lessens with standard treatment.

At this point, pain is no longer a symptom, and it has become an illness, triggering a series of emotional, physical, and social consequences that become a real scourge, not only for the person suffering from the pain, but also for the people in their lives.

In these situations, pain can appear suddenly. It can be produced by normally harmless stimuli, a phenomenon known as "allodynia," in which pain is produced by pressure as light as touching your bedsheets. Alternatively, exaggerated and prolonged painful reactions to a recognized harmful stimulus is called "hyperalgesia." When this occurs in locations other than the site of the primary wound it is called "secondary hyperalgesia."

On a physiopathological level are several mechanisms that we can explain as they chronicle pain. It is necessary to first explain sensitization, which is a phenomenon whose principal function is to reinforce the protective function that occurs after being exposed to intense stimuli repeatedly. These stimuli make sure that the nerve endings responsible for receiving painful sensations (nociceptors) are activated by less intense stimuli (decreasing the activation threshold) and that the response produced by the stimulation will be greater (amplified response). The sensitization, therefore, is an adaptive response and makes sure the body is alert to these situations in which the probability of injury is high. Once past the period of danger without injury, this exaggerated sensitization disappears, the body returns to normal, and the nociceptors require more intense stimuli for activation (normalization of the activation threshold).

When this phenomenon continues over time and loses its protection function, that is to say, the feeling remains after the incident of injury, it becomes one of the most important mechanisms to explain how pain becomes chronic.

At this point, it is necessary to understand the concept of "neuronal plasticity" that consists of the capacity of the nervous system to remodel the contacts between the neurons to adapt to different situations. If we use terms derived from materials science, and specifically related to the properties of these metals, it would be a kind of malleability that these nerve cells possess in order to adjust to the different changes to which they are subjected. This phenomenon, the same as sensitization, has a protective character and occurs habitually after a nerve injury when the other neurons adapt to meet the functional deficiencies caused by the injured nerves.

Sensitization can occur both peripherally (located in the nerves within the skin, muscles, etc.), or at a central level (located in the brain and spine). Previously, it was believed that chronic pain originated at the central level, and that peripheral sensitization simply had a secondary role; now, there are studies that show that the peripherals have a greater role in this phenomenon.

It is known that peripheral sensitization occurs after the exposure of the peripheral nociceptors to substances derived from inflammation or tissue damage, and causes painful hypersensitivity in the inflamed area (primary hyperalgesia). It was previously believed that this pain would stop once the stimulus disappeared. Now it has been demonstrated that on the peripheral level, neuronal plasticity mechanisms can occur by which nociceptors respond exaggeratedly to an acute inflammatory aggression, or to a stressful environmental event. The injured tissue becomes a receptor that only responds to harmful mechanical stimuli (high threshold mechanoreceptor), to a receiver that responds to non-harmful stimuli (low threshold mechanoreceptor).

This is their function at the level of clinical practice where we know that many chronic pain conditions can be initiated by one or more transient acutely painful episodes. Experimental studies on rats have tried to identify which is the mechanism that produces this event and they have failed to demonstrate that an acute painful event can predispose a later phase of hyperalgesia. In this event, it is related to an enzyme known as the protein kinase C in its isoform Epsilon (PKC-e).

There are conditions that can be predisposed to prolonged hypersensitivity. For example, the repetition of painful movements can cause safe movements to be painful as well. Also, stressful environmental conditions can trigger a state of persistent hyperalgesia.

This has been shown in studies conducted on mice, in which those subjected to stressful noisy environments suffer from hyperalgesia more often than those who are not exposed to this stressor (it is important to highlight that the hyperalgesia is indistinguishable from the reaction produced by inflammatory mediators). At the same time, it is demonstrated that stress by itself is capable of increasing levels of inflammatory substances that contribute to hyperalgesia.

Hypersensitivity on a peripheral level, both derived from tissue damage and from other causes, can condition sensitivity on a central level that is without a doubt the principal mechanism of the production of chronic pain and explains how functional, structural, or biochemical changes produced in the medula and brain produce abnormal pain sensitivity. The neuronal plasticity is determined by the occurrence of central sensitization, the changes in the neurons that produce a change in function. These can exist in the cellular level where there is increased excitability of the membrane covering these cells, improving efficiency of communication between neurons (synaptic improvement) or decreasing the activity of the inhibitory neurons (there is less inhibition of transmitted signals). The net effect of all these phenomena is a state of facilitation, potentiation, or amplification of the painful stimulus.

Understanding the mechanisms of the production of the central sensitization is essential for understanding the physiopathology of common painful syndromes such as neuropathic pain, migraines, irritable bowel syndrome, fibromyalgia, etc. In these patients, an abnormal response to harmless stimuli occurs, there is hypersensitivity beyond the site of the injury, the system for interpreting the pain is altered and does not distinguish between harmful and harmless stimuli. If we understand this pain generation mechanism we can find direct treatment to relieve this state of hypersensitivity. This is the great challenge of current medicine.

For over twenty-five years, there has been scientific evidence that central sensitization is involved in the genesis of chronic pain. Clifford J. Woolf, using an animal model, was the first scientist to demonstrate that the continuous repeated application of painful stimulation is capable of generating functional changes at the level of the spinal cord (revisiting the concept of neuronal plasticity). His work consisted of administering heat that caused moderate inflammation in the area of application, and then a harmless stimulus was applied to the area outside the injury where it produced a painful response. More recent studies have demonstrated changes not only to the spinal cord but also to other cerebral areas.

We must remember that in order to produce the central sensitization, it is necessary to create a prolonged, constant, intense stimulus. And that this does not produce the activation of a single nerve transmission pathway; also, a large number of molecular processes are necessary for its development. The most important functional changes that can be found in the neurons affected by central sensitization are: the generation and growth of spontaneous activity, the lowering of the activation threshold, and the growth of the field receptor stimuli. These changes are produced by three mechanisms: growth of the excitability of the membrane, facilitation of the synaptic efficacy or decrease of the inhibitory signals.

The changes that happen at a molecular level clearly escape the objectives of this book. Nevertheless, we believe that we must make a quick reference to what happens on this level in order to understand a little about the different medical treatments. The most important are changes in the number, threshold, and activation of cell receptors called NMDA (N-methyl D-aspartate) and AMPA (alpha-amino-3-hydroxy-5-methyl-4-isoxazolepropionic) that are dependent on an amino acid with a function activity with other known inhibitory receptors such as GABA (gamma-aminobutyric acid) and the production of glycine, which is an amino acid inhibitor. This is what, in the end, produces the aforementioned facilitation of synapses, increase in excitability of the cellular membranes, and disinhibition of the neurons.

Despite great advances that have been made in learning about where chronic pain comes from, and all the molecular processes that have been discovered, there are still many things that are not clear. If we understand these mechanisms we can formulate specific treatments and improve the quality of life of the people who suffer from this serious problem. The development of new technologies and the progress in research create a hopeful future.

Psychological Consequences Associated with Chronic Pain

Dr. María Teresa Vicente, Dr. Luis Aliaga

Pain is a perceptual process whose impact on personal life depends on a variety of factors, such as the patient's state of mind, environment, social support, and economic resources. The medical practice demonstrates that pain is frightening to patients when its source is unknown. A diagnosis can help facilitate the acceptance of pain and diminish suffering.

One model that best explains the experience of chronic pain and the relationship with other chronic problems associated with this is the biopsychosocial model.

CHRONIC PAIN AND DEPRESSION

Scientific studies concede that a person who suffers from chronic pain is more likely to suffer from depression and anxiety. According to the study *Pain in Europe*, Spain exhibits the highest percentage of depression associated with pain of any country in the European Union. One out of every ten Spanish citizens suffers from chronic pain, which directly affects one in four families. And

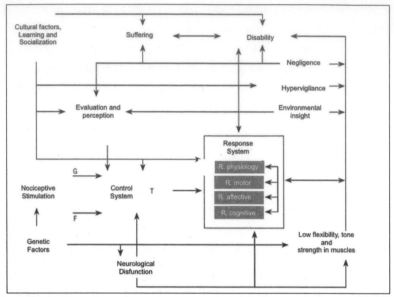

(J. Miró. 2003)

29 percent of those affected suffer from depression as a result of being in pain day after day. Depression is not the only emotion that accompanies chronic pain; it is also common to experience anxiety, guilt, irritability, and confusion.

There is a greater percentage of depressive symptoms in patients with chronic pain than in the general population or among others suffering from chronic illness. They are the most susceptible to suffer from depression than before if they had few activities, few sources of satisfaction, and few skills. And they feel the most vulnerable if they believe that what they do will not help anything.

Depression has been understood as a negative response to one's illness. Nevertheless, as Professor Ricardo Manzanera from the Imperial College of Medicine in London points out, the manifestation of pain is a common symptom of depression.

Other symptoms include disordered sleep, sexual problems, fatigue, and loss of appetite. These symptoms can be treated with different painkillers and anti-inflammatories with poor results which also mask the underlying depression and can produce serious side effects, complicating the evaluation of the patient.

From the available facts it is possible to come to the conclusion that depression is caused by a deficit in neurotransmitters, namely noradrenaline and serotonin, which play an essential role in controlling moods and pain. This deficit provokes a decrease in the pain threshold since the inhibitors do not work properly.

With the appearance of tricyclic antidepressants and their widespread use in the treatment of depression, it was found that these drugs relieve pain in the context of the depression. This gives root to the theory that chronic pain is linked to emotional disorders. Currently, the data supports that both depression and pain have common neurobiological mechanisms.

It is important that patients freely analyze the implications of the proposed treatments and make decisions related to their treatment with family members and a doctor. Research shows that these depressive feelings confirm the psychological suffering and increase the pain, establishing a vicious cycle. That is to say, we are faced with not only a medical issue but also a biopsychosocial issue as well. And this is how it should be treated. It is not enough to treat pain medically, but it is necessary to use psychological therapy. Unfortunately, despite the existence of plenty of studies that demonstrate its effectiveness, psychological therapy is infrequently applied.

There are two schools of thought when it comes to pain treatment. One proclaims "it is all in your head" and the other argues that "it is all in your body." Nevertheless, one study coordinated by Chantal Berna, from the University of Oxford, shows that pain is an amalgam of both. According to her research, when a person is sad or depressed, this destroys the skills used to regulate negative emotions associated with pain, provoking a greater pain reaction or greater suffering. Likewise, both anxiety and irritability negatively influence the perception of pain.

THE SOCIOECONOMIC IMPACT OF PAIN

As to the socioeconomic consequences, specialists say that pain can have a considerable impact on the lives of those suffering from pain, as well as on their families. Nineteen percent of people affected by chronic pain have lost their job as a consequence of this pain, and 16 percent have had to change their occupation. Pain is the cause of more than fifteen days off a year in the European Union. This, along with the expected progressive aging of the population, in the coming years, will produce and increase in the prevalence of chronic musculoskeletal pain because of their relationship with degenerative pathologies. At the same time, the economic and social impact of this situations requires innovative approaches for conducting diagnostics on pain and the efficacy of current treatments. Herein lies the importance of pain clinics, which we will discuss later.

THE ROLE OF PSYCHOLOGY IN PAIN TREATMENT

Psychology offers various resources that can help treat pain as an illness. Patients can make changes in their daily life that can improve their attitude about their pain. This is why it is so important to include a psychologist on staff at pain clinics. Psychology offers valuable information to other doctors and members of the staff as well. This interdisciplinary approach to pain treatment is helpful to a team cooperating and contributing to understanding the psychological impact of pain on a patient's life.

In fact, many patients are surprised when they are referred to a psychologist to treat chronic pain, as they had perceived their illness as purely physical. Nevertheless, as we have previously explained, pain is often affected by a patient's psychological state, which is introduced to the patient with phrases like, "We want to understand how pain influences your life," or "we want to help you get better." Indeed, the psychological treatment of chronic pain has shown to have a great impact on the patient and their social environment. In this sense, any information that helps a patient's family is very useful. In addition to one-on-one meetings between the patient and a psychologist, it is also important for the psychologist to meet in groups with the patient's friends and family members to give the doctor a better picture of the patient's everyday life.

Group psychological treatment among patients suffering from chronic pain has advantages, because it allows for the patient to talk with others experiencing similar problems. This can help reduce stress and feelings of isolation and disability. It is also useful to learn about what kinds of strategies other patients use to help handle their pain. In addition to group therapy that requires a psychologist to lead the discussion, there are other support techniques that can help alleviate chronic pain.

The evaluation and treatment of chronic pain should focus on the individual, rather than the pain itself. In the following tables, we outline the goals of psychological assessment and treatment of patients with chronic pain.

Objectives in the psychological evaluation of patients with chronic pain (J. Miró, 2003):

- Evaluate the patient's history with pain
- Learn which treatments the patient has sought out and their effects
- Identify the level of physical function prior to the onset of the problem
- Learn about the patient's own theories of what causes their pain.
- Establish the patient's current level of physical activity
- Clarify the advantages and disadvantages that are caused by chronic pain
- Identify the the psychosocial factors associated with chronic pain
- Differentiate the causes and effects of the problem
- Establish objectives for treatment
- Create an outline for a customized program according to the needs and characteristics of the patient
- Evaluate the current progress during and after the treatment
- Examine the patient's satisfaction with the treatment in contrast to the evaluated progress
- Assess the satisfaction of the family members with the treatment and progress of the patient
- Track the patient's progress
- Reconceptualize the problem of pain. Try to help the patient think of pain as a manageable problem, eliminating feelings of hopelessness
- Teach the relationship between thoughts, feelings, and actions, and their effect on a physical level

- Help the patient take an active role in the resolution of the problem, teaching them that they are a competent person with resources to solve problems
- Teach the patient coping mechanisms and problem-solving skills that can be used to improve their quality of life
- Promote expectations of personal effectiveness and positive self-esteem, in relation to the results achieved during treatment
- Help the patients to prevent relapse, anticipate problems and find solutions
- Facilitate the maintenance of results obtained during the treatment program

COGNITIVE-BEHAVIORAL THERAPY TO TREAT PAIN

Among psychological therapies, the most studied are those called "cognitive-behavioral." Patients treated with cognitive-behavioral therapy show a decrease in pain, anxiety and depression, providing increased activity and quality of life.

Before we get to the different techniques that constitute this branch of therapy, we should explain the patients, and how their emotions and behaviors can increase pain. The goal of therapy is to learn how to understand and control emotions and actions. This understanding will help the patient during their therapy. Let's look at the most common techniques used to fight pain.

BREATHING AND RELAXING

Breathing is said to be the first approach a patient can use to control their pain, and is the first step in methods to help with relaxation, breaking the circle of anxiety-pain-anxiety. Relaxation, even though it is not in itself therapy, can be learned by the body and mind. Its greatest benefit is that it helps the patient control their psychophysical activity and perception of pain while increasing their vitality and feelings of control and balance, which can help fight depression and anxiety. Relaxation reduces muscle tension which can contribute to pain. The first step is to explain this vicious cycle to patients. That is to say, how pain creates tension, which in turn increases pain. Once a patient learns how to relax, they are encouraged to practice these techniques on their own.

BIOFEEDBACK

The use of biofeedback (BF) is relatively new. It began to be employed in the 1960s. The objective of this technique is to learn to control the physiological response related to a particular clinical problem. The patient uses an electronic machine that monitors their physical functions, letting the patient see and hear what is happening in their own body. Depending on the type of physiological response that they see, the patient can learn what stimulates certain activity in their heart, in their muscles, change in temperature, etc. In this way they can learn to control their response. The use of BF has been well documented in chronic pain treatment. Many studies have demonstrated its efficacy in the treatment of tension headaches, cluster headaches, migraines, neck pain, temporomandibular pain, shoulder pain, back pain, myofascial syndrome, rheumatoid arthritis, pain from cancer, and phantom limb pain. The efficacy of BF is due to both the control of the physiological response, as well as the ability of this treatment to modify other variables implied in the treatment of chronic pain. These variables are primarily cognitive-attributional as expectations of improvement, self-efficacy expectations, or the perception of control. The capacity of BF to modify these variables is not often taken into account, despite having an important influence on the overall effectiveness of the treatment.

- **Care Management:** If pain is distracting us, it will increase and cause more suffering. We can learn to control our attention, and keep it off of the pain.
- **Cognitive Restructuring:** To a greater or lesser extent, we all distort information, that is to say, we are all biased. This form of biased thinking can manifest in what is called "catastrophic thoughts" ("I can't go on," "I am useless"). There is a distinct correlation between catastrophic thinking and pain. The objective is to help the patient recognize and understand these different distortions that can cause us to think in these exaggerated ways.
- **Solving Problems:** Developing skills to help solve problems can help us to have a less stressful life. In the case of patients with chronic pain, stress can increase pain. We can apply techniques with the objective to teach patients to define their problems and identify possible solutions.
- **Emotional Management:** The first objective is for patients to learn to identify what emotions they feel, in which circumstances they feel them, and why. That is to say, patients learn to be self-aware in order to help control the emotions that contribute to their pain. The second objective is to improve the relationships with themselves since in many cases, pain can fog the mind.
- **Values and Setting Goals:** First, the patient reflects deeply on the most important values in their life. Next, they establish specific goals to make improvements. This is to try to translate all the reflections on their life into concrete objectives to achieve through therapy.
- **Time Management:** People who suffer from pain need more time to complete certain activities. Because of this, they

eliminate many fun activities from their schedule in order to get their errands done. In this part of therapy, the patient learns better ways to organize their time in order to be able to still make room for social activities and hobbies.

- **Physical Exercise, Posture, and Sleep Therapy:** It is necessary to emphasize the importance of physical exercise, and discuss the possible barriers that patients may encounter. It is also important to work on posture and sleep therapy to improve these aspects of a patient's life in order to help reduce pain.

INSOMNIA

From a clinical perspective, there is a strong relationship between chronic pain and insomnia as experiencing pain can make it difficult to get to sleep and stay asleep. One of the most studied variables that causes insomnia is depression. The presence of depression caused by chronic pain can contribute to high prevalence of sleep disorders. In fact, studies have shown that sleep disorders are more closely correlated with severe depression than with pain.

Sleep disorders can also be caused by taking pain killers. Opiates and corticosteroids can influence the sleep cycle and NSAIDS have also had different effects on sleep.

The first step a patient needs to take to treat their chronic pain and insomnia should be to evaluate their symptoms. They need to find the right sleep clinic, observe their sleep and waking patterns, their family history of sleep disorders, and previous treatments, before considering a diagnosis of insomnia.

The Placebo Effect

Dr. María Teresa Vicente, Dr. Luis Aliaga

A "placebo" is a substance or strategy without any medical value which nevertheless produces a curative effect when consumed by the patient. The placebo effect is a phenomenon that can help improve the patient's symptom.

"Placebo" is a Latin word from the verb *placere* (to please), conjugated to the first person singular future, meaning "I will please," a translation which holds the secret of its current meaning. When someone believes that the drug or procedure will improve their condition, it is more likely that their condition will improve

The term "placebo" was first used in a medical context in the first half of the twentieth century, coinciding with the creation of drugs with demonstrable healing power. Around this time, doctors were using antibiotics to cure illness effectively, and studying the effects. In contrast to these effective drugs and the scientific examples, certain drugs and treatments were showing results without any scientific proof. They named these substances "placebos." Before modern medicine developed drugs with therapeutic effects, that vast majority of medicine used until then (ointments, medicinal plants, salves, etc.) were showing effects due to the placebo effect. But they were not simply placebos: they were substances that despite having no medical value, still produce curative effects.

Now, the placebo effect is not only recognized scientifically but also used for research. It is curious that the term "placebo" appeared at the same time as active drugs, and at the same time, the scientific determination of drug efficacy is proven by contrast placebos. We have read, for example, on the data sheet for Viagra: "During the research study more than 3,700 men tried Viagra. [. . .] Between 60 and 80% of the results were positive, in comparison to the 25% of patients who had success with the placebo (a sugar pill)." The study demonstrates that the placebo has equal effect as the Viagra does on one in four men.

Aside from the role that placebos play in today's clinical trials, scientists have been interested in researching the healing effects of placebos. In the year 2000, the American National Institute of Health conducted a study called "The Science of Placebo." Since then, there have been many publications on the subject.

Current technology has identified the area of our brain that, when activated by the placebo effect, produces endorphins, which create a similar effect to morphine and help to relieve pain. This activation is the final part of the complete process and still is not sufficiently studied. In this sense, together with the suffering and pain that frequently accompanies illness, we realize that the situation is psychologically complex and reveals as many internal factors as external. Among patients, their previous education may influence their response to pain. Much remains to be studied about these conditions. Surely, this field of study sheds much light on chronic pain.

Before man understood and used the placebo effect, it was observed in everyday life. Many world literature texts offer a description of the placebo effect. The following passage is from Charmides (one of the Dialogues of Plato): "The remedy was a kind of grass that works when used with a certain incantation, but without that incantation is useless." Plato recognizes that the secret lies in the incantation that needs to go along with the grass, which is precisely a placebo.

Many other literary references demonstrate the existence of the placebo effect across time. In *Don Quixote*, for example, we find a reference to the famous balm of Gilead, which Don Quixote explains as "a balm whose recipe I know by heart, which will cure any fear of death or any mortal wound." Cervantes talks about the science of the placebo effect. It doesn't matter what the recipe is for the balm: what is most important is that the patient believes in its healing effects. And it is not only a cure, but can also resuscitate the patient: "and, with this balm, if you see that I have parted from my body during battle (which is known to happen), or if I have lost a limb, give me two but two drops of this balm and you will see me become sounder than an apple."

More recently, but no less illustrative, from the seventeenth to twentieth centuries, references continue in different passages of *The History of San Michele*, the autobiography of the doctor Axel Munthe, which alludes to the best qualities of a doctor—inspiring the confidence of his patients or, similarly, helping them to find the self-reliance to improve their health—"I looked not to the patient, but to his family member. It was a serious case. The patient's pessimism had infected the entire house; the patient was paralyzed with discouragement and fear of death. It was probably that my two colleagues understood pathology better than I did, but I knew something that they were ignoring: that there is no drug more powerful than hope." And we continue reading: "I had the luck, surprising luck, almost magical [. . .]. No doubt I was a successful doctor. But what is the secret to my success? In the case of a doctor, without a doubt: inspire success. The doctor that can do this will be able to resuscitate the dead."

And, finally, among many other possible references, we found a story published in 1961 called "Shadows in the Grass" (a continuation of the great novel *Out of Africa*), a passage from the autobiography of the baroness Karen Blixen, who recorded her experience trying to treat the pain of a badly injured boy in the jungle: "It is a sad experience to sit by somebody suffering so direly without being able to help. . . . In my distress I once more put my hand into my pocket and felt the King's letter. 'Yes, Kitau,' I said, 'I have got something more. I have got something very excellent indeed. It is a thing which people known, that a letter from a king, in his own hand, will do away with all pain, however bad.' And I laid the King's letter on his chest and my hand upon it. I endeavoured, I believe, out there in the forest, where Kitau and I were as if all alone, to lay the whole of my strength into it [. . .] It was a very strange thing that almost at once the words and gesture seemed to send an effect through him [. . .] I was almost surprised when he spoke to me: 'Yes,' he said, 'It is excellent,' and again, 'yes, it is excellent. Keep it there. . . . You will sit beside me and hold it to my stomach as before, or otherwise the bad pain will come back at once.'" The rumor of the amazing healing effect of the letter spreads among the sharecroppers on the farm, and they ask for it as a remedy ("they demanded to borrow the King's letter, for the day or for the day and night, to take with them to the hut for the relief of an old dying grandmother or small ailing child"). The author concludes: "The King's letter amongst my stock of medicine from the very first was accurately and strictly placed in a category of its own. This decision was taken by the Natives themselves without my giving any thought to the matter. It would do away with pain, in this capacity it was infallible, and no ache or pang could hold out against it."

In short, the placebo effect has been well demonstrated and has been used by doctors as a therapeutic tool. When scientific pharmacology began to become a reality, it was considered that it was no longer necessary to continue struggling, wasting time.

Listening calmly and patiently, or making sure you are put together when talking to the patient, are all ways to reassure the individual and inspire confidence.

In recent years, it has been demonstrated why those amazing results have been described in universal. Fortunately also for patients, the placebo effect has piqued the interest of scientists. It has been demonstrated that placebos help reduce habitual doses of pharmaceuticals. We can conclude that doctors should make sure they listen to their patients, and give them encouragement. It is important to make sure patients remain hopeful and open to curing their illness. It is necessary, above all, to consider all aspects related to placebo effects as part of the big picture related to treating chronic pain.

Pain Clinics

Dr. Antonio Ojeda, Dr. Carlos Nebreda, Dr. Luis Aliaga

From the end of last century, great progress has been achieved in regard to understanding the physiopathology of pain, and substantial improvements have been made in diagnostics and treatment of chronic pain. Likewise, the necessity to create specialized treatments for each patient has been accepted. From these developments, pain clinics were born.

Professionals can work on offering their patients the best possible individualized management for their pain. Pain treatment has become a new subspecialty of medicine.

Pain clinics are organizations that work towards the prevention, diagnosis, treatment, research, and understanding of pain. They are staffed with specialists who offer a multidisciplinary approach to treating the root of the pain. The attention that these specialists can provide are based on constantly updated knowledge. Pain clinics are well equipped to apply the newest therapies and techniques for treating pain safely and effectively. The clinics earn their accreditation by implementing systems for quality control in order to ensure efficiency in all areas of work.

The fundamental objective of the pain clinics is the integral attention paid to the patients in order to help improve their quality of life, and restore their physical well-being, as well as their social and emotional lives. The majority of people visiting a pain clinic do not have a cure for their underlying illness, and the treatment they receive at the clinic will help them relieve their symptoms.

The treatment of chronic pain focuses not only on the physical treatment of pain, but also on the psychosocial plane. In order to help the patient in all aspects, it is necessary to treat the psychological and psychiatric symptoms and the problems that occur in their social life derived from this pathological process. Therefore, it is fundamental that the pain clinics have trained staff, whether clinical psychologists, or psychiatrists with experience treating chronic pain.

During the 1950s, Dr. John J. Bonica became the first doctor to implement the concept of multidisciplinary pain treatment. His idea came from observing the treatment of patients with difficult symptoms, and how the process of referring these patients to multiple specialists was a cumbersome, slow, and ineffective process.

It has been shown that multidisciplinary evaluation and multimodal treatment substantially improves the life of patients suffering from chronic pain. Dr. Flor and his collaborators conducted a meta-analysis (scientific study that analyzes the facts from other medical publications), in which it was shown that multidisciplinary and multimodal evaluation is better than unidisciplinary and unimodal treatment of chronic pain. In this study, it was found that patients that were given multidisciplinary treatments reduced their consumption of pharmaceuticals, and 60 percent were able to return to work, while of the group being treated with unidisciplinary methods, only 30 percent of the patients were able to return to work.

It was also shown that the pain assessment from a multidisciplinary pain clinic is cost effective. That is to say, it is cheaper for the healthcare system, as the patients not only visit fewer specialists, but they also visit them with less frequency. Also, the patients have a greater chance of recovery, which improves their social environment.

The importance of multimodal treatment (for example, pharmaceuticals combined with meditation or psychological treatment) has been shown in many studies on the resolution of pain, with the majority of patients returning to work after suffering from migraines, arthritis, and back pain.

WHEN SHOULD YOU VISIT A PAIN CLINIC?

Patients who visit a pain clinic are a group of very different people. Many of the patients are referred by other specialists and already have a physical diagnosis to explain their pain. In this case, they are seeking advice on how to manage their pain and control their symptoms. Other patients do not have a specific diagnosis. In these cases, serious physical causes should be excluded by the doctor, as this type of patient is suffering from a psychological issue. Another group of patients are those who visit a pain clinic to receive diagnostic nerve blocks in order to intervene on future attacks. One example of the use of diagnostic nerve blocks is on the lumbar facet joint before the radiofrequency of the nerve involved in the origin of the pain. That is to say, the first objective in finding the cause of the pain is to locate this nerve and next to find a more aggressive treatment.

Waiting too long to receive an assessment of chronic pain can lead to a disability that was potentially preventable. Referral to these specialized clinics should not be a last resort.

There is a publication that reviews the different opinions of professionals involved in pain treatment in the United States, where it has been observed that the best time to refer a patient with chronic pain to a pain clinic is within 8 months. On the other hand, the North American Spine Society has considered that the referral must be made within 4–6 months after the beginning of pain with severe symptoms and evidence of physical and psycho-social deterioration.

Despite the diverse typology of patients who are visiting a pain clinic, we try to classify them in three groups to be evaluated by a multidisciplinary unit specializing in pain. In one group, we have patients with persistent pain with a known cause, and without suc-cessful treatment, in which the results of measures taken are insuf-ficient and the pain is interfering with their daily activities and energy levels.

In the next group, we have patients with consistent pain and an unknown cause, but for whom very serious causes have been excluded. And, finally, we have patients whose pathologies can benefit from a short visit to these, such as patients of post-herpetic neuralgia, cancer pain, complex regional pain syndrome, reflex sympathetic dystrophy, phantom limb pain, or back pain, among others.

In all of these cases, pain clinics are capable of improving the medical, psychological, and socio environmental aspects of the patient's life. At the clinic, doctors are able to work as a team to revise their methods, using the patient's history and previous expe-riences, in order to develop a specific plan for the treatment of the patient. They can also create methods to help educate the patient on each step of the process.

Pain clinics help evaluate patients and achieve results. Once the pain is under control, the treatment can be continued with the patient's family doctor.

It is important to emphasize that pain clinics are not remote and inaccessible, and a last resort for patients, but instead should be visited early on in treatment.

PHARMACOLOGICAL TREATMENT OF PAIN

In the previous chapter, we saw how human beings have employed an endless number of therapies to try to alleviate pain. In ancient civilizations, they used plants whose tranquilizing ingredients have been isolated and are used in present day medicine (e.g., opium, morphine, aspirin).

It is necessary to note that these painkillers do not work for all kinds of pain, but depending on the characteristics and the form of production (pathophysiology), a patient will be given a particular drug. For example, pain caused by a nerve injury (neuropathic pain) does not respond much to non-steroidal anti-inflammatories (NSAIDs), or pain caused by muscle contraction will not be alleviated by opiates (morphine, etc).

We also want to underline that all pharmaceuticals have many adverse side effects, and must be prescribed by a professional. Self-medication presents a great risk to patients.

NON-STEROIDAL ANTI-INFLAMMATORIES (NSAIDS)

NSAIDs are commonly found in medicines, like painkillers, antipyretics (for the treatment of fevers), or anti-inflammatories. They are made up of very chemically heterogenous group of drugs that have one principal mechanism in common: the decrease in inflammatory mediators called "prostaglandins" through the inhibition of the enzyme cyclooxygenase (COX). The use of the expression "non-steroidal" is to differentiate between very strong anti-inflammatories like corticosteroids. The original and most widely studied NSAID is acetylsalicylic acid (aspirin). Other commonly known NSAIDs are ibuprofen, diclofenac and dexketoprofen. They have multiple side effects and must be used with caution by patients with heart, kidney, digestive problems, or bleeding disorders, who can be predisposed to the development of renal failure, high blood pressure, heart attack, gastric ulcers with perforation and bleeding, etc. Patients should also be cautious of allergic reactions and hematological problems.

PARACETAMOL (ACETAMINOPHEN)

Paracetamol (acetaminophen) is one of the most commonly used medicines in the world to treat pain and fever, and is the medicine most prescribed to children. It is used as a painkiller for light to moderate pain. Its pharmacological characteristics give it its own place in pain treatment. It does not have anti-inflammatory properties and it is not effective for pain caused by smooth muscle spasm (colicky pain). Unlike NSAIDs, it is not harmful on a gastrointestinal, renal, or cardiovascular level. Despite its widespread use, its active mechanism continues to be a mystery. It was previously proposed that its principal mechanism was related to the inhibition of inflammatory mediators in the central nervous system (prostaglandins). And, while it is true that a decrease in the levels of these substances occurs in the brain, it has recently been postulated that its most important mechanism of action is produced by the indirect activation of cannabinoids. It is a safe drug at therapeutic doses, with the maximum adult dose of 4 grams a day. Problematic side effects are rare, but have shown an increase in liver transaminases, hypotension, hypersensitivity reactions, and blood disorders. An overdose can cause severe liver failure.

OPIATES

Opiates are excellent painkillers, and are used to treat moderate to severe pain. They are effective in treating pain that results from specific receptors located both in the central nervous system and peripheral nervous system. By their degree of affinity to these receptors, they are classified as pure agonists, partial agonists, or agonist-antagonists. The first include the most commonly used, among which is morphine. Other drugs in this group are hydromorphone, codeine, oxycodone, methadone and fentanyl. Opiates have many side effects: constipation, nausea, vomiting, urinary retention, confusion, sedation, and respiratory depression. These effects vary in frequency and severity depending on the prescribed drug. The partial agonist most commonly used is buprenorphine, while the most common agonist-antagonist is pentazocine. People who are prescribed pure agonists should not also be prescribed an agonist-antagonist because this can trigger a withdrawal syndrome or increase pain.

OTHER PRESCRIPTION PAINKILLERS
There is another group of frequently used painkillers: co-analgesics and interveners. Co-analgesics are medicines that were not originally created for the treatment of pain, but due to its pharmacological properties, they are can be used to alleviate pain. Interveners help treat symptoms that affect patients suffering from pain, such as insomnia and depression.

ANTIDEPRESSANTS
Antidepressants are not only used by chronic pain patients to improve their mood, but they are also used as painkillers themselves and can enhance the effects of other drugs, like opiates. Their painkilling actions are created through the increase of substances that control pain (above all, noradrenaline). Antidepressants are effective in treating neuropathic pain caused by diabetic neuropathy or postherpetic neuralgia.

Among this group of drugs are tricyclic antidepressants (amitriptyline, clomipramine). They have been widely used in clinical experience. Although their effectiveness has been proven in many clinical studies, its possible side effects require that they be used with caution in certain types of patients (cardiac patients, the elderly). Also, they sometimes cause intolerance in many people, limiting their use. Nevertheless, the side effect profile can sometimes be helpful. For example, amitriptyline can improve the sleep habits of patients suffering from insomnia.

One relatively new group of antidepressants are serotonin reuptake inhibitors (fluoxetine, paroxetine) and the dual inhibitors of serotonin and noradrenaline (duloxetine, venlafaxine). These drugs have the advantage of fewer side effects, greater safety profile (they can be used with cardiac patients or the elderly) and they have similar efficacy in regard to the treatment of depression as tricyclic antidepressants. Nevertheless, the majority of these are less strong than tricyclic antidepressants. They include the growing role duloxetine plays in the treatment of generalized pain syndromes such as fibromyalgia.

It is necessary to note that these drugs do not act right away. They usually take about one or two weeks to show results. During this period the patient may experience side effects without improving their symptoms. If the patient continues to feel these side effects, doctors recommend that the patient continue taking the medicine as the side effects typically disappear after a few days.

ANTICONVULSANTS

As its name indicates, anticonvulsants were initially used for the treatment of epilepsy. Today they have become one of the fundamental treatments for neuropathic pain. Its primary mechanism consists of the suppression of abnormal nervous stimuli. In this group of drugs, standouts include: carbamazepine, which has been the drug of choice for a long time for the treatment of trigeminal neuralgia; gabapentin, which has been used with great results to treat numerous symptoms of neuropathic pain (like post-herpetic neuralgia, diabetic neuropathy, neuropathy associated with HIV or Reflex Sympathetic Dystrophy) and also has found decreased allodynia and hyperalgesia associated in patients suffering neuropathic pain; and pregabalin, which is a new anticonvulsant that has generated great interest in recent years, that has basically the same effects as gabapentin but a better safety profile and only needs to be taken twice a day instead of three times.

Anticonvulsants also have many side effects, like lightheadedness, drowsiness, fatigue, and weight gain. As in the case of antidepressants, they do not take effect immediately, but a patient may need to wait one or two weeks before they see results.

ANXIOLYTICS

Anxiety is one of the most common symptoms of chronic pain. While sometimes psychotherapeutic treatment is enough to treat this symptom, it is also sometimes necessary to use specific drugs. The best prescription drugs for the treatment of anxiety are benzodiazepines (diazepam, clonazepam, lorazepam, etc.). Among these, clonazepam stands out for its results in treating aches and muscle pain. These drugs should be used with extreme caution with children and elderly patients, people with muscle disorders, and people with breathing problems. They also increase the risk of increasing tolerance (needing to increase the dosage constantly to create the same effect) and developing a physical and psychological tolerance. It is necessary to be careful when using these with central nervous system depressants like opiates, as they can enhance the appearance of respiratory depression.

CORTICOSTEROIDS

Corticosteroids are a medication with great anti-inflammatory power. They are effective in treating cancer pain, especially headaches from brain tumors (produced by the increase in intracranial pressure secondary to peritumoral edema), bone pain, and pain caused by spinal or nerve compression. Its possible side effects include the increase in sugar levels in the blood (hyperglycemia) above all in diabetic patients, arterial hypertension, production of gastric ulcers, and, in the case of chronic treatment, the production of osteoporosis, the suppression of the production of corticosteroids or Exogenous Cushing syndrome.

MUSCLE RELAXERS

Muscle relaxers are typically not used for chronic treatment, but can quickly help to relieve muscle contractions related to AECB especially produced in patients that suffer from myofascial pain syndrome (painful muscle contractions). Cyclobenzaprine and tizanidine stand out in this group. Also included in this group are benzodiazepines, which in addition to their effect on relieving anxiety, they also act as a muscle relaxer.

BISPHOSPHONATES

Bisphosphonates are drugs that act by inhibiting bone resorption and have been effective in alieving pain caused by cancer that has invaded the bones (bone metastases).

THE WORLD HEALTH ORGANIZATION'S PAIN LADDER

During the first half of the twentieth century, pain went unobserved for most global associations linked to health. In the 1980s, concern for this issue became more prevalent, since it was estimated that more than 50 percent of cancer patients were not adequately treated. This led many of the greatest specialists to meet and decide to create a simple method to apply simple and effective treatment for cancer patients suffering pain. In 1986 (after a preliminary version in 1984) *Cancer Pain Relief* was published.

The World Health Organization's (WHO) Pain Ladder consists of a three-step ladder that aligns the treatment plan with the pain intensity level. The first step is for patients with light to moderate pain, for which the use of NSAIDs and paracetamol are recommended,

The second step is for the use of "weak or lesser opioids," which include codeine, tramadol, and dextropropoxyphene. And the third step is for stronger opioids, for the treatment of intense pain; this group includes morphine, fentanyl, methadone, oxycodone, etc.

Regardless of the intensity of pain, you can add adjuvant drugs, which are drugs that can help diminish pain by acting differently from the aforementioned drugs. Among this group are antidepressants, benzodiazepines, bisphosphonates, local anesthetics, anticonvulsants, etc.

In the document, the WHO also recommends the following pillars for pharmacological treatment:

1. Drugs should be administered orally.
2. Drugs should be administered at regular intervals ("by the clock"). This allows for continuous pain relief. If the patient continues to have pain with this regimen, it is possible to monitor when and how pain reappears, if it is associated with a certain activity, or comes out of nowhere. An appropriate dose of the medication can be adjusted.
3. The pain ladder should be used when possible.
4. Attention must be paid to detail. That is to say, careful attention to the patient and their family, their full drug regimen, and all the side effects.
5. Individualized treatment should be given to each patient.

Studies have been done that show that different forms of this protocol outlined by the WHO have shown 70–90 percent efficacy.

Even though this has been a very important step in treating pain, there are cases where the application of this protocol is not always appropriate. For example, the steps are not enough to treat pain from lung disease, postoperative pain, or acute pain. Also, depending on the patient's disease, sometimes taking oral medicine is not appropriate. In severe cases, this can delay the patient from getting proper treatment.

Some specialists add a fourth rung to the ladder, including interventional techniques used in cases like peripheral nerve blocks, alternative techniques for drug delivery, and neurosurgical techniques such as neurostimulation.

In 2002, the Spanish Pain Society (SED) established the concept of the elevator for pain treatment. In this protocol, the different drugs and treatments are on different "floors," and there are four buttons in the elevator representing the intensity of the patient's pain. The first button is for light pain: treated with NSAIDs, paracetamol, and metamizol. The second, moderate pain: weak opioids. The third, intense pain: strong opioids. And the fourth floor, unbearable pain: specialized units. In this metaphorical elevator, there is also an "alarm button" for when the intensity of pain is extremely high (as a fifth rung on the pain ladder). This elevator concept involves an immediate response to the patient's pain, without establishing a phased order.

INTERVENTIONAL TREATMENTS PERFORMED IN PAIN CLINICS

Pain clinics count on qualified specialists to create diverse techniques that allow them to help patients who suffer from pain, and who have not achieved results through regular use of painkillers. According to the American Society Of Interventional Pain Physicians, interventional treatment of pain has the goal of diminishing and managing pain and improving the quality of life of the patient, through minimally invasive techniques specifically designed to diagnose or treat various pain syndromes.

With increased medical knowledge and safety of the techniques used, more patients are returning to daily activities, their pain is decreasing or disappearing, as is their need for routine pain medications. Next, we summarize some common interventional techniques.

PERIPHERAL NERVE BLOCKS

Pain is transmitted by nerves located in different regions of our body. A nerve block prevents the passage of these pain signals to the central nervous system. Local anesthetics are used to treat this pain. Different techniques are used to locate the nerve or nerve plexus, including neurostimulation (stimulating the nerve with electricity creates a motor response that allows the patient to pinpoint the block), and x-rays, which allow patients to locate difficult to see nerves directly, or through understanding the surrounding anatomy.

EPIDURAL STEROID INJECTIONS

Epidural Steroid Injections are particularly suitable for radicular pain due to irritation or inflammation of a nerve root. It is a very common procedure that consists of the placement of corticosteroids in the epidural space often accompanied by local anesthetics. It can be performed through radiology, or blind. A drug is injected adjacent to the nerve that is causing the pain.

JOINT PAIN

The most common locations of joint pain are in the shoulder, hip, knee, and sacroiliac joint (located at the bottom of the spine, which is responsible for 15 percent of back pain). Joint pain is typically treated with local anesthetics and steroids. Its effectiveness is greater if performed with x-ray visualization.

INFILTRATION OF THE FACET JOINTS OF THE SPINE

Infiltrations are used in the diagnosis and treatment of back pain that comes from the facet joints in the spine. Facet joints connect the vertebrae. When they are affected by different pathologies, like arthritis, this can produce mechanical lumbar pain. Direct vision radiation (fluoroscopy) is used to locate these joints in order to be able to administer local anesthetics and corticosteroids into the joint (intra articular lock) or the nerve next to the damaged joint. This technique is often used as a diagnostic tool to determine the origin of the pain. If it works, it can be seen as a treatment specific to its pathology, and the nerve endings responsible for transmitting this pain.

TRANSCUTANEOUS ELECTRICAL NERVE STIMULATION (TENS)

Transcutaneous Electrical Nerve Stimulation is the administration of an electrical current by placing electrodes on the skin of the affected area. This current selectively stimulates peripheral nerve fibers that can block the transmission of pain impulses to the brain (according to the theory of the gateway). This is a non-invasive technique that is easy to apply and has few side effects. The joints directly link to improve the uptake of ionizable substances used for the treatment of pain, which are usually corticosteroids and local anesthetics. It is a painless and safe treatment and can be useful in treating painful chronic illnesses like back pain and osteoarthritis.

INFILTRATION OF TRIGGER POINTS

This technique is employed for the treatment of myofascial pain (painful muscle contractures). This consists of the infiltration of a medicine (local anesthetic or a corticoid) in the places whose palpation box triggers the patient muscle pain (trigger points), allowing them to block the painful stimuli and producing muscle elongation (relaxation of groups of tense muscles). Sometimes, the infiltration may be performed with saline or can even be done without liquid (dry tap), a painless and simple technique. It takes five to ten minutes depending on the number of trigger points found.

RADIOFREQUENCY

Radiofrequency is a method based on sending low-energy high-frequency electrical currents through two electrodes. One of the electrodes (the active electrode) is insulated along its entire length except for the tip, and it is used to address the treated area. The other electrode (dispersive electrode) is a plate of conductive material with a larger uninsulated area than the active electrode. The passage of a current through this circuit generates heat at the tip of the active electrode to perform treatment.

Depending on how this heat is administered, two types of radio frequency can be derived. Traditional radiofrequency uses temperatures higher than 150 degrees Fahrenheit, producing neuron injury, and is a painful process. Pulsed radiofrequency, on the other hand, uses temperatures below 113 degrees Fahrenheit, inducing changes along the neuron membrane or production of chemical mediators that block painful stimulus without causing injury. Depending on the use and type of the pain, one or the other technique is recommended.

Examples of how RF can be used include: the treatment of trigeminal neuralgia, lumbar pain (especially facet syndrome), cervical syndrome (cervicogenic headache, facet syndrome, cervical-brachial), intercostal neuralgia, intractable malignant pain, or lumbar sympathectomy. Radiofrequency of peripheral nerves can help in the treatment of painful syndromes in certain areas (occipital nerves, suprascapular nerves, femoral cutaneous, intercostal, etc.).

REGIONAL SYMPATHETIC BLOCKS

In certain illnesses, pain is mediated by the sympathetic autonomic nervous system. In these cases it is necessary to block these nerves to control pain. The treatment is usually performed under direct visualization with the help of radiology and local anesthetics. Occasionally, for long term treatment, the block can be caused by drugs (chemical neurolysis) or temperature (radiofrequency thermocoagulation). The most common blocks used in treatments are for stellate ganglions, celiac plexus, and hypogastric plexus, among others.

IMPLANTABLE DRUG INFUSION SYSTEMS

There are a number of patients with chronic pain who have shown a good response to analgesic drugs but, because of side effects and other circumstances, cannot take them through the common methods (oral, transdermal). In these cases, they can place the drug dose near the site of the pain's source. Through a minor surgical procedure, a small device consisting of a reservoir pump and a small catheter can be inserted in the area by the spinal cord (intrathecal space), where the nerves that transmit pain are located. Putting the drugs right in the place of action allows for a significant decrease in dosage. For example, intrathecal morphine is three hundred times more potent than morphine taken orally. This allows for the greater control over the pain with fewer side effects.

IMPLANTABLE NEUROSTIMULATORS

In certain patients with difficult to treat chronic pain, or in those for whom the side effects of common pharmaceuticals are intolerable, implantable neurostimulators are a good alternative for pain relief. A small apparatus is implanted under the skin, that emits electrical signals to an electrode just below the nerves that transmit pain signals. This blocks the pain signals and helps alleviate pain. The main causes for this treatment are failed back surgery, complex regional pain syndrome, or untreatable angina, among others.

BOTULINUM TOXIN INFILTRATIONS

The botulinum toxin is a neurotoxin produced by a bacteria called clostridium botulinum. It is used to block the release of acetylcholine, which is necessary to contract muscles. Preventing muscle contraction is useful for the treatment of painful myofascial syndromes, like piriformis syndrome or the psoas muscle.

HOMEOPATHY AND CHRONIC PAIN

The word "homeopathy" comes from the Greek *homo* (similar) and *patia* (suffering). It is an alternative method based on the theory that "like cures like" and that a greater dilution has a higher power. This method is the opposite of allopathy, which says that symptoms should be treated with chemicals that oppose the manifestation of the same.

For many years, they have tried to elucidate the true effect of this form of alternative medicine. Even today, there are still questions surrounding its effectiveness. Scientific works exist that prove that homeopathy is no more effective than placebos (substances that lack therapeutic action) for the treatment of illnesses.

Nevertheless, there are reports that this kind of medical practice can be useful in the treatment of chronic pain, such as migraines, fibromyalgia or rheumatoid arthritis.

The most important study done on this subject was published in the prestigious medical journal *Lancet* in 2005. The study was done with over 110 clinical subjects in which no evidence was found that the homeopathic treatment was more effective than the placebo.

The authors of this study report that any improvement in patients treated with homeopathy is more related to their experience with therapy than with homeopath, as this treatment dedicates more time and attention to the patient than conventional medicine.

As to chronic pain and homeopathy, there are many references. As for the treatment of other diseases, there are people who advocate this type of medicine and people who disagree. As we previously mentioned, there are reports that it may be useful in the treatment of fibromyalgia, migraines, and trigeminal neuralgia and rheumatoid arthritis. Nevertheless, the majority of these works are lacking in references to the applied scientific method. There is a recent study published about the efficacy of homeopathy in the treatment of fibromyalgia. In this study, there is not significant evidence found that this therapy is effective for the treatment of this illness.

In spite of what has been published, there remain several points of view surrounding this type of alternative medicine. So, the debate, far from being settled, remains as open in the field of medicine based on evidence, as on the non-medical publications.

Natural Solutions to Common Pains

Dr. Luis Aliaga, Carlota Máñez

If something hurts, the priority is clear: stop the pain. For this, the majority agrees on using analgesics and anti-inflammatories. When the pain does not stop, one may ask to go to the doctor and learn about the causes of what is bothering them so badly. It is true that sometimes medicine can help at first, stopping the pain without finding the cause can cause problems later on. For example, if we take a painkiller at the first sign of back pain and then continue with everyday life (exercise, hours in front of the computer, etc), the pain will become even worse. If we take the time to figure out the cause of the pain, we can act accordingly and cause many more benefits: the pain can go away as well as whatever was causing it.

The first advice that we give to someone disposed to follow a natural treatment to a health problem is that they need to understand that the primary objective of natural medicine is to regain balance in all aspects of a person, not only to attack the painful symptoms. Another difference between conventional medicine and natural, is the mental attitude of the patient. Conventional medicine relies on pharmaceuticals, which only requires a passive attitude on the patient's part, which is to say that the patient takes the medicine and then they do nothing else to fight their pain.

Natural medicine requires the patient to act. Phytotherapy, following acupuncture, is fundamental to help fight your pain, but it is also necessary to take care of your health, paying attention to what your body is trying to tell you.

There are many ways to fight different kinds of pain and their causes. Some of these therapies and techniques that we will explain can be administered and applied by oneself, while others require the supervision of a specialist in conventional or alternative medicine.

Pain has become an important part of patient care and is actually considered, together with temperature or arterial tension, to be a vital sign. Chronic pain can negatively affect a patient's entire physical state including the psyche of the patient and their quality of life. It is a complex factor influenced not only by the illness it creates, but also in terms of psychological aspects, past painful experiences, the environment, and the genetics of each individual.

We must also consider the marketing, that is, people do what is most touted without it being an actually effective treatment. Also, natural medicine is not without side effects or pharmacological interactions.

Alert System

Pain can act as a messenger for when our body is not working correctly. In this sense, it can act as a friend or an enemy. And that is apart from being an alert system against aggressions of different kinds, and also can act as a mechanism of aggression when it persists (chronic pain), changing the quality life and making every day activities difficult. As to the intensity, the pain can be light, moderate, or severe, and in general is conditioned by the disease it causes. Nevertheless, the way pain manifests itself has a lot to do with the attitude of the patient. A relaxed perspective can help control pain more easily.

Chronic Pain Increases Risk of Falling for the Elderly

According to the study from the Beth Israel Deaconess Medical Center in Boston (US), that was published in the Journal of the American Medical Association (JAMA), older people who suffer from chronic musculoskeletal pain in two or more locations, primarily in the shoulders and knees, besides those with more severe pain that interferes with their daily activities, are more likely to fall than other individuals.

The analysis of the data revealed that, in comparison with the participants in the study who claimed to not have any pain, those with chronic pain in two or more joints had up to a 50% increase in their risk of falling. So, the authors of this study suggest that pain can be added to the list of factors involved in the risk of falling and that the people who have chronic pain in two or more joints and who suffer from moderate to severe pain are at a higher risk.

PAIN IN RHEUMATIC DISEASES

Even though many people frequently use the term "rheumatic pain" especially to describe those vague, transitory pains related to weather changes, this definition is not used by health professionals. Rheumatic pains are actually those that affect the locomotor or musculoskeletal systems, integrated by bones, muscles, tendons, joints, connective tissue, and ligaments.

According to a study done by the Spanish Rheumatology Society (SER), almost one in four Spanish adults suffer some rheumatic illness, representing 22.6 percent of the population, and more than six million people are taking anti-inflammatories for treatment, which provoke gastrointestinal complications in about a third of patients.

Without the use of drugs, people are finding other natural solutions for treating this type of pain. It is necessary to realize that practically all patients suffering from rheumatic pain are in pain at any moment. A specialist can help control this symptom rather than treating the illness, while doctors tend to put the pain in the background, while handling each specific rheumatic case.

In recent years, we have seen important advancements in the understanding of the mechanisms that produce and regulate pain sensations. Specifically, among the mechanisms that produce rheumatic pain and how it is influenced by the joint inflammation and the psychological state of the patient.

"Even small changes in the intensity of the pain can affect the patient's outlook," explain the authors of an article about rheumatic pain that was published recently in the magazine *Arthritis & Rheumatism*.

PHYTOTHERAPY

The use of medicinal plants in the different treatments of inflammatory reactions, in particular, in osteomuscular pain, have increased effectiveness and are believed to have several advantages compared to common anti-inflammatories, such as lower likelihood of side effects. Joint pain, back pain, lumbago, gout, rheumatism or more specific ailments such as muscle pulls or sprains can be fought with certain medicinal plants, some of which are the base for various medicines. One of these is aspirin, originally derived from willow bark, which is a clear example of the contribution that plants have made in modern science.

One of these natural alternatives to non-steroidal anti-inflammatory drugs (NSAIDs), drugs that often cause stomach problems, is Harpagophytum, or devil's claw. Thanks to this healing plant, commonly found in the Kalahari Desert in South Africa, those who suffer from this pain can avoid having to choose between their stomach and their knees.

- **Devil's claw** (*Harpagophytum procumbens*)

According to the Center for Phytotherapy Research (INFITO), devil's claw is a therapeutic option that is effective in treating pains related to musculoskeletal inflammation and, what is even better, without the undesirable side effects caused by traditional treatments. Different studies show the efficacy of this plant for its anti-inflammatory action, as an antirheumatic and analgesic in the treatment of chronic polyarthritis, lumbar degenerative joint diseases and muscle pain, in the shoulder and back, light or moderate.

Devil's claw stops the action of cyclooxygenase, responsible for pain and inflammation in rheumatic illnesses, as do common anti-inflammatories. Its painkilling and anti-inflammatory function is due to the joint activity of its active ingredients (harpagoside).

It is frequently ground up and taken in capsules, which helps eliminate its bitter flavor, and it is much more agreeable and practical to take when prepared this way. It is also common to use the dried and chopped root to prepare decoctions and fluid extract (1.5 ml every 8 hours). It can also be used with other anti-rheumatic plants to prepare infusions.

Do not use if you have a peptic ulcer, gastritis, or biliary obstruction. It is also not recommended when pregnant or breast-feeding, or for small children.

> *Antirheumatic maceration:* Pour 4.5 g of the devil's claw root into a container with 300 ml of water and let sit at room temperature for 8 hours. Strain and drink throughout the day in 3 sittings.

&. *Tisane for arthritis and gout:* Mix one part willow, one part java, and two parts devil's claw. Mix one teaspoon of this mixture into a cup of boiling water and let sit for 10 minutes. Strain and add honey to sweeten. Drink three times a day, after a meal.

- **Canadian horseweed** (*Erigeron canadensis*)

This plant, which Native Americans have always used for their medicines, is noted for its diuretic and anti-inflammatory effects. For this reason, it is used as a remedy in the treatment of rheumatic diseases and arthritis, effectively alleviating inflamed joint pain.

In addition to its anti-inflammatory action, it prevents gout and its diuretic action contributes to the reabsorption of edemas and retention of liquids.

The plant can be found, dried and ground, ready to prepare infusions (two teaspoons per cup), or for decoctions and in extract form (1–2.5 ml every 8 hours). Nevertheless, it is most commonly used in the form of capsules, and the recommended dose is indicated by the manufacturer.

&. *Infusion for rheumatic pain:* Mix one tablespoon of the dried plant in a cup of boiling water. Let sit for 10 minutes and strain. To relieve joint pain, you should take three cups a day, one after each meal.

&. *Combined with devil's claw and black currant:* This enhances its efficacy to alleviate rheumatic pain. Do not use if pregnant or breastfeeding, or for small children.

- **Ash** (*Fraxinus excelsior*)

Ash, or European Ash, is traditionally used to fight muscle and joint
pain. It has not only been demonstrated to have anti-inflammatory
virtues but also diuretic effects. This
facilitates the removal of substances
such as urea and urate through
urination. It is often used as a natural remedy to fight painful inflam-

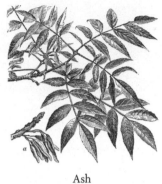

Ash

mation. Increasing urination is also helpful in avoiding edemas
(retention of liquid) and preventing kidney stones.

It is most frequently found ground in capsules (the dose
is indicated by the manufacturer) even though it is possible to
acquire the plant dried and chopped for preparing decoctions
(10–30 g per liter of water; take one or two times a day), in extract
form (0.5–1.5 ml every 8 hours) and in tinctures (2.5–5 ml every
8 hours).

> 🐾 *Infusion to alleviate rheumatic pain:* Mix equal parts
> ash, black currant, nettle, meadowsweet, and java. Mix
> one tablespoon with one cup of boiling water and let sit
> for 10 minutes. Strain and drink one cup every 8 hours.
> This alleviates rheumatic pain and pain associated with
> gout.

- **Black currant** (*Ribes nigrum*)

Even though it is well known for its delicious black fruits, in phytotherapy, black currants are appreciated for their medicinal virtues
and their leaves, which are diuretics and anti-inflammatories. Among

other uses, they are traditionally used to relieve pain and inflammation produced by insect bites.

The leaves of the black currant plant play an important anti-inflammatory and anti-rheumatic role, without the inconveniences that allopathic medicines can have. The anti-inflammatory effect, linked to its potent diuretic action that helps eliminate waste like urea and uric acid, allows for this remedy to also be used in treating gout, as well as

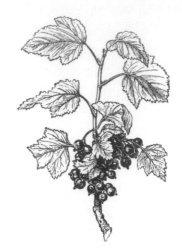

Black Currant

to increase diuresis in genitourinary disorders such as cystitis.

The leaves are most commonly found dried and sliced, ready to be used in infusions (2–4 g per cup of water). It is also used in capsules (the dosage is indicated by the manufacturer) and in syrup (5–10 ml every 8 hours). Also, it is included as a diuretic and anti-inflammatory in many mixtures. The fruits are most commonly found fresh or in the form of juice.

> 🌿 *Diuretic infusion:* Put two or three teaspoons of the dried leaves in one cup of boiling water. Let rest ten minutes and strain. Taking one cup several times a day increases diuresis which helps alleviate rheumatic discomforts.
>
> 🌿 *Diuretic infusion to alleviate joint discomfort:* Mix equal parts of dandelion, black currant, and rampion. From this mixture take one or two heaping tablespoons and boil with one cup of water. Let rest ten minutes and strain. Take three cups a day, after meals.

Black currant leaves should not be used if you are pregnant, breastfeeding, or for small children. In case of kidney or heart failure, or hypertension, you should consult a specialist before use.

- **White willow** (*Salix alba*)

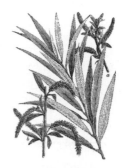

White Willow

This plant was used for centuries in China, ancient Greece, and medieval Europe. Native Americans have also used this plant to treat headaches, fevers, and muscle pains. In 1882, salicin was extracted from the plant, a substance that was soon purified into salicylic acid. This is effective in treating pain and fever, but also for removing warts, and was subsequently modified (this time from anthemis, to create salicylic acid, the primary active ingredient in aspirin.

Salicin has antipyretic, analgesic, antirheumatic, and antiseptic properties. It is an excellent natural remedy to treat mild febrile illnesses. It is also effective to treat rheumatic pains in muscles and joints, back pain, and tendinitis.

As interest in natural medicine grows, white willow has begun to be considered as an alternative to aspirin. Willow bark is part of antirheumatic treatments, most commonly in capsules and mixed with the devil's claw root. It is also frequently found in mixes for infusions to treat colds and flu.

You can find it on its own, dried and ground for decoctions (two teaspoons per cup of water), in extract form (1–2 ml every 8 hours), and in tinctures (5–8 ml every 8 hours). It is also found in capsules, with the dosage indicated by the manufacturer.

You should not use this if you have gastritis, peptic ulcers, asthma, an allergy to salicylates, coagulation disorders, or for children under sixteen years old. It is also not recommended if you are pregnant or breastfeeding.

White willow bark is considered a good alternative for aspirin.

- *Analgesic decoction:* Combine one or two teaspoons with one cup of water and boil for a few minutes. Let sit for five minutes and strain. This can be taken up to four times a day, preferably with meals.
- *Decoction for pain:* Mix one part yellow chamomile flower, one elder flower, and two parts white willow bark. From this mix, take two teaspoons and mix with water, and boil for a few minutes. Let sit for 15 minutes then strain. Take 2 cups a day, after meals.

- **Meadowsweet** (*Filipendula ulmaria*)

Also known as "queen of the meadow," this beautiful plant has been used since the sixteenth century to treat rheumatic pain. Like the willow bark, it was used for salicylates extracted from it with its antipyretic properties (to lower fevers) and from which aspirin was derived. In fact, the name "aspirin" comes from its Latin name: *Spiraea ulmaria*.

When metabolized, some of its principal actions are transformed into salicylates, with anti-inflammatory, antipyretic, and analgesic properties. But it also has a marked diuretic effect that facilitates the elimination of uric acid and urea. Because of this, this remedy is used to treat muscle and joint pains and gout. It is also an effective recourse for treating flu and fevers, and to avoid edemas (liquid retention) and prevent the formation of kidney stones. Likewise, it has an anticoagulant effect that helps prevent thromboembolism, but should be used with caution if you are being treated with other anticoagulants.

It is mainly used with other plants, in preparations (mixes for infusions, capsules, and tablets) used with antirheumatics. But you can also find it on its own, dried and ground for infusions (one teaspoon per cup of water), in extract (2–3 ml every 8 hours), and in tinctures (2–4 ml every 24 hours).

It is not recommended for patients who are allergic to salicylates, have peptic ulcers, gastritis, or who are pregnant or breastfeeding. It is also not recommended for children. If you have asthma or clotting disorders, consult a specialist before taking it.

For the treatment of rheumatism, it can be combined with devil's claw, black currant, and willow bark.

> 🍂 *Antirheumatic infusion:* Combine 1 teaspoon of dried flowering tops and one cup of boiling water and let sit for 10 minutes. Strain and take after meals.
> 🍂 *Decoction for external use:* Combine 25g of meadowsweet with 1 liter of water and boil for 15 minutes. Strain and use in a bath (no longer than 10 minutes) to alleviate joint and muscle pain.

- **Oregano** (*Origanum vulgare*)

Commonly used in cooking, oregano is known to restore appetite and prevent flatulence. But when used externally, it is effective in relieving joint pain and certain postural discomfort such as torticollis. It is converted into essential oil and the drops are applied to the painful area and massaged in two or three times a day. For a toothache, you can boil two table-spoons of oregano with poppy and two cloves for five minutes, let rest for another ten minutes. Rinse your mouth well with this mixture several times a day.

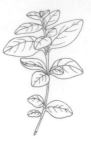

Oregano

> **Also . . .**
> Other plants used in the treatment of muscle, rheumatic, and osseous pains are viburnum (*Viburnum opulus*), primrose (*Primula veris*), marjoram (*Origanum majorana*), and basil (*Ocinum basilicum*).

HOMEOPATHY

This therapy can provide significant relief from pain and prevent the disease from continuing to develop.

Homeopathy is one of the most common alternatives for people who prefer to avoid conventional drugs. Homeopathic medicine "cures like with like" and uses products from animals, vegetables, and minerals, which in high doses cause the same symptoms in a healthy person as the patient, while curing the patient. In this way, the *Coffea* remedy (coffee) can cure insomnia, while *Allium cepa* (onion) is made from vegetables and minerals. It is a therapy created by the German doctor Samuel Hahnemann, and has been used for over a century. The difference from conventional medicine and allopathy is that those work by treating symptoms with their opposite. For example, antibiotics are used to kill bacteria.

Treatment should be individualized for each patient, but common remedies are: Byronia, Pulsatilla, Causticum, Rhus tox and

Ruta graveolens, depending on which kind of pain you are trying to treat.

ACUPUNCTURE

Acupuncture can also have very effective results and produce lasting benefits. The method and technique help mobilize energy, drain stagnant fluids, heat cold parts of the body, and cool down others.

EXERCISE

The benefits of exercise are clearly demonstrated in patients of chronic osteomuscular pain. Regular activity improves muscle tone and stabilizes the musculoskeletal system. Physical exercise increases the production of endogenous opioids (endorphins) that reduce pain. It also improves mental health and wellbeing.

However, a sedentary life is as harmful to our bones as excessively aggressive sports and can cause arthritis and annoying fractures, and encourage potential falls. The best exercise for bone health is called isometrics or progressive resistance, based on small doses of intense activity, like moderate running, walking, and dancing. The six most recommended physical activities are:

- **Water aerobics**: The resistance of the water helps develop muscle strength, flexibility and balance.
- **Jogging:** Increases muscle bone density in the spine and hips. To be effective, it is best not to practice two days in a row. Patients should begin a very gentle program and gain intensity progressively. This helps fight arthritis and osteoporosis.
- **Tai-chi:** Excellent for developing balance, strengthening the legs and improving flexibility. Reduces muscle tension from stress and improves focus.

- **Weight training:** Improve resistance with small weights and many repetitions. To improve muscle mass, it is preferable to lift small amounts of weight, many times, very slowly. It is important not to lift too much weight.
- **Jumping rope:** Improves bones in the hips in premenopausal women. Simply, jump rope for a minute to increase strength in the calves, and improve balance. Jumping rope is helpful in fighting osteoarthritis in the spine, legs and hips.
- **Dancing:** An activity that because of its impact on the floor can help with bone growth and improve patients' moods.

A sedentary life is as just as bad for our bones as aggressive sports.

REFLEXOTHERAPY

This technique of therapeutic foot massage is very old, and has been known to be used in China for five thousand years, and in Egypt for the past four thousand. The theory and map that therapists in the West use were developed in the 1930s by the American physiotherapist Eunice Ingham. She considered the feet to be reflective of the entire body, and, as they are one of the areas of the body with the most nerve endings, it is possible to stimulate and activate different organs. The objective of this therapy is to encourage the body to regain balance. First, the patient is given a foot massage and then certain areas are focused on using different techniques.

It is believed to be very beneficial to illnesses in the musculoskeletal system, except for in cases of osteomyelitis (bone infection) and cancer. It can accelerate recovery from a fracture or break, improve osteoporosis, stimulate organs that help in the absorption of calcium, and diminish pain from fibromyalgia.

HYDROTHERAPY

Water is an excellent way to mediate temperature. This thermal effect is good for the bones. Baths and hot tubs are effective ways to treat one's body with water. Exercising in water is also effective, especially to help recover from a trauma. It is helpful to alleviate inflammatory or degenerative diseases, such as osteoarthritis. It is also a great way to treat joint problems.

OZONE THERAPY

Ozone therapy is more of an alternative method without proven effects, than a natural therapy. It is used to treat many painful illnesses: from osteoarthritis in multiple joints (especially knee, spine, shoulder, etc.) to fibromyalgia and lumbar pain related to intervertebral disc disease. It is believed to have important anti-inflammatory power and reduces important free radicals that perpetuate the inflammatory process. Ozone is injected in the affected joint in the form of mixed gas. It has few adverse side effects, although there are records of certain cases of gas embolisms that can compromise the life of the patient.

CLAY AND HOT WATER BOTTLES

These are useful to alleviate pain that is produced from bone decalcification. Gentle massages with analgesic plants are also advised.

STRESS RELIEF

Stress creates major muscular tension and increases pressure between bones. It also diminishes the capacity to absorb calcium. Relaxing activities like yoga and tai-chi not only reduce stress but are also beneficial to bone and muscle health.

DIET

Diet is the most important part of the foundation for repairing and maintaining bone, muscles, and connective tissue. The lack of certain nutrients can provoke demineralization with serious consequence like osteoporosis. It is important to follow a balanced diet with lots of vitamin D and calcium. Vitamin D can be found in cod liver, blue fish, egg yolks, milk, and butter. The daily dose can be easily achieved with 20 g of tuna. Get 15 minutes of sun a day on the face and hands, and this should be enough vitamin D. The recommended dose of calcium is 800 mg a day (found in milk and other dairy products). It is important to have 2 to 4 servings of milk and dairy a day (one serving is about one cup of milk, two yogurts, or 50 g of cheese). Other sources are almonds, sesame, leafy green vegetables, small fish with bones (sardines, anchovies, etc.).

Connective tissue helps maintain the structure of the body, especially cartilage, tendons, and ligaments in the joints. To strengthen and regenerate the connective tissue, it is important to take care of your joints. The best natural antioxidants for this are curcumin, powdered bamboo to regenerate bones, borage oil rich in linolenic acid, and manganese. Vitamins A, B, C, D and E (anti-inflammatories and antioxidants), magnesium maintains bones and joints, papain and bromelain, and papaya and pineapple extracts, are especially recommended to help with joint pain and stiffness.

Collagen hydrolyzate (gelatin) helps improve the function of collagen, the principal component in cartilage. Collagen is a protein that surrounds certain organs to protect them and maintain elasticity in the tissue. It is indispensable in all cases and it is necessary to contribute to the maintenance of the cartilage tissues. Clinical studies show that the daily administration of hydrolyzate at the recommended doses over two months improves symptoms in patients in the first stages of osteoarthritis, and the motor skills of patients with chronic osteoarthritis.

MENTAL THERAPY

Relaxation, meditation, and hypnosis are therapies that reinforce pain-relieving impulses sent from the brain. The effectiveness of these methods has yet to be proven scientifically. Massage and transdermal nerve stimulation are complementary therapies to be applied by a professional.

MANUAL THERAPIES

Although there is little scientific evidence to back them up, treatments like massage, acupuncture, osteopathy, and other techniques applied with hands are defended by many as a way to relieve spinal pain.

Caution with Opioids

Pharmaceutical opioids are the strongest painkiller that we have. Although their classic use is to treat pain from cancer, their use has extended with success to treating other kinds of chronic pain.

In fact, in musculoskeletal pain, we have seen an increase from 8 percent to 16 percent in patients prescribed these drugs in the last 20 years.

Opioids like morphine or codeine are often prescribed, or synthetic drugs like tramadol.

There is still little experience in the use of these drugs for chronic rheumatic pain. The potential to develop addiction and dependency is problematic for doctors.

It is also true that this type of treatment, while a good way to control pain, can also increase the care a patient needs as they are powerful sedatives.

HEADACHES

It has been calculated that six in every ten people in developed countries suffer from frequent headaches. The most pessimistic studies affirm that almost 90 percent of the population in developed countries suffer from tension headaches, which is a very common syndrome. It has also been noted that women suffer from this problem more than men. Another type of headache is the cluster headache, which is more frequently found in men, and is considered to be more serious. They affect only 1 percent of the population. The stress of modern life seems to be behind this progressive growth of the incidence of headaches.

Curiously, the vast majority of headaches do not originate in the brain. In reality, more than 90 percent of headaches begin in the muscular fibers and in the blood vessels in the scalp and neck. Some causes of pain in this zone can be from muscular contraction (from stress, for example), whiplash (from a fast and sudden movement of the neck), or irritation of the nerve endings provoked by chemical substances like alcohol, tobacco, or inhalation of gases.

Types of Headaches
- **Tension:** This is the most common kind of headache, affecting many more women and most people have suffered from this at some point in their lives. It is caused when muscles in the head and neck contract from a physical cause (many hours in front of the computer or a strain), or emotional cause (stress, anxiety, depression). When the muscles contract, they press on the blood vessels keeping them from transporting oxygen to the tissues. The tissues, deprived of the oxygen they need, release the neurotransmitters related to pain (histamine, serotonin, etc.).
- **Food:** One of the most important factors that contributes to a headache is food. For example, it could be that

you are allergic to an ingredient or product, and this can affect the sugar level in the blood causing a headache. Caffeine, aspartame (artificial sweetener), chocolate, MSG (flavor enhancer found in processed foods), cheese, and dry fruit, are all foods whose consumption is related to frequent headaches. Also, lack or excess of certain vitamins or minerals can be the cause of many headaches: low levels of copper or magnesium, lack of vitamins B6, B12, and folic acid, or excess of vitamin A, a growing problem among people who take supplements without medical supervision.

- **Tobacco and Alcohol:** Tobacco is a vasoconstrictor, and can easily cause headaches. Alcohol also has effects of vasodilators but when consumed in excess, the toxins can produce a headache.

- **Hormonal Imbalances:** Many headaches in women can be traced back to imbalances in two principal hormones: estrogen and progesterone. The most common is produced by an imbalance in the patient's estrogen level. The increase of estrogen during premenstrual syndrome can cause fluid retention, which can provoke a headache. Upon arriving at menopause, the drastic reduction of the level of estrogen is precisely what causes headaches. Headaches can also be related to taking contraceptives that contain estrogen and progesterone.

- **Environmental Factors:** Noise, pollution, chemicals from cleaning products, dyes, or weather—all of these factors can cause headaches. Allergies to pollen, dust, mites, fur, and mold can also cause headaches, as well as light and smell.

- **Sports:** Any sport practiced in excess can produce a headache, from overexertion. Sports that can cause headaches the most are diving, jogging, and weightlifting.
- **Hypertension:** Hypertension itself does not cause headaches; nevertheless, when a patient shows elevated numbers suddenly, this can trigger what is known as "hypertensive encephalopathy." Many people with hypertension claim to see that they have headaches when they wake up but the pain goes away a little after taking their medication. It is easy to see that the pain is caused in moments of stress (when the tension increases) or if a patient eats very salty food (which also increases tension).
- **Sleep Habits:** It is important to note that lack of sleep—a very common problem—can cause headaches and other pains.
- **Vision Problems:** Spending hours in front of the computer (for work or other reasons) or in front of the television, using glasses with the wrong prescription, and so on are all frequent causes of headaches. Glaucoma (an eyeball disorder that is characterized by an increase in intraocular pressure) is a serious health problem that can also cause headaches.
- **Organ Disorders:** Headaches can often be caused from poorly functioning organs (intestines, liver, etc.).
- **Taking Medicine, Neurological Problems, and Vertebral Column Problems:** These are other factors that can trigger a headache.
- **Cluster Headaches:** These are often related to the sudden release of histamine or serotonin from tissues. It has also been found that they may be related to the excessive

consumption of alcohol, which directly affects the blood vessels and the nerves.

- **Neuralgia:** This is a headache caused by the irritation of a nerve. One of the most common is caused by the inflammation of the trigeminal nerve (or pain in the face), which descends from the side of the face, or causes sensitivity in the face, mouth, teeth, nasal cavity and the muscles in the mandible. It can limit important movements related to chewing and talking. This is considered to be one of the worst pains that can be suffered. It is a very sharp headache and can be short but often repeated. It impedes on talking or chewing normally and is more often found in women than in men. This pain can be produced in different areas, depending on different nerve endings. The first trigeminal nerve is in the front of the eye, the second, the maxilla, the third, chin and lower jaw.

- **Migraine:** This type of headache affects almost 12 percent of the American population. Its primary symptom is a strong headache in one or both sides of the skull. It is different than other headaches because it is often accompanied by digestive issues (nausea, vomiting), and hypersensitivity to environmental stimuli (light, sound, and smell). In 85 percent of cases, it is preceded by an aura, a series of neurological symptoms that indicates a transient dysfunction in part of the brain, which can last about ten minutes. The aura is most frequently visual (flashing lights, darkening vision, image distortion . . .). Migraines can repeat in several attacks between 4 and 27 hours, which can be an incapacitating pain. Even though the symptoms are the same between most patients, the causes for each individual's migraines can be very different. There is a strong hereditary component, and hormonal changes in women can be a very important factor (thus, this has come to be seen as a woman's illness). Other factors causing migraines include: liver, kidney, or bladder dysfunction, stress, and long-term abuse of alcohol or drugs.

Natural therapies consider the existence of sick people rather than diseases, because the therapies they offer are completely personalized. Specialists examine both the migraine symptoms and the characteristics of each individual person to identify a treatment that is unique and different for every patient. At first, these therapies, as with conventional medicine, also help find relief for the migraine symptoms, but after various sessions they try to discover the internal imbalance of the patient in order to help heal their entire body.

TRADITIONAL CHINESE MEDICINE

To reestablish equilibrium within the body, some natural therapies focus on the flow of energy (Chi) that circulates through the body and whose alteration is the suspected cause of many migraines. Traditional Chinese medicine, which explains migraines as the result of dysfunction among the internal organs, especially the spleen, liver, and kidneys in addition to an emotional disorder. To treat it, specialists first locate the pain, crossing each organ's meridians: pain from the vertex area is from the liver; in the temples, it is from the vesicles; and when found around the eyes, it is from the liver and stomach.

If pain is felt most strongly in the morning, it represents a major deficiency in Chi, and if it is worse at night it is because of a lack of Xue (blood). The most recommended method of treatment for this is acupuncture, which is based in the insertion of fine needles in the skin following the channels through which energy circulates to return its flow to normal. It is very effective when paired with phytotherapy or Tui Na massage, which uses fingers instead of needles.

SHIATSU

Shiatsu is a therapeutic art that works on the body following the meridians and points described in traditional Chinese medicine; this method uses pressure from the thumbs and hands and also uses elbows, knees, and feet. Basically, it tries to promote fluid movement of vital energy, channeling the excess energy from other parts of the body and moving it to where it needs to go. Normally the specialist begins with the liver, the vesicles, the heart, and the bladder (these are the meridians that should be treated if you suffer from migraines) to help find relief that at first will only be symptomatic.

YOGA AND MEDITATION

The mind plays a greatly important role in the beginning of feeling pain: the fear of suffering a new crisis can provoke anxiety and trigger the episode. Because of this, relaxation techniques like meditation and yoga are very effective tools in taking the necessary mental control to prevent pain. These are techniques that can help in crucial moments, but also can be practiced regularly to help understand and eliminate physical and mental tensions that often provoke migraines.

HOMEOPATHY

The sensation of pain changes the character of a person, as they live with the fear of a new attack, the mere thought of which can trigger more pain. This point is considered by homeopathy specialists, who consider the particular characteristics of each patient in order to find the most sensible remedy. The most common remedies are: Natrum muriaticum and Ignatia for migraines due to emotional factors; Sepia and Actea Racemosa for migraines produced by hormonal changes; Nux Vomica or Pulsatilla in migraines related to digestive or liver disorders; or Belladona for migraines caused by circulatory issues.

REFLEXOTHERAPY

This technique is achieved by the proper handling of the soles of the feet, for the purpose of detecting illnesses and contributing to their cure. This therapeutic foot massage is not only a treatment but also a diagnostic method, so the specialist can discover in which organ the problem is located by pressing on special zones.

DIET

Food can help explain certain migraines: prolonged fasting, large meals, consumption of alcohol (especially red wine), the ingestion of vasoactive amines (chocolates, cheese, dry fruit, bananas, sausages, etc.) and of additives such as MSG (commonly found in precooked foods and Chinese cuisine) and nitrites or nitrates (used in meat products like sausages, foie gras, etc.) are recognized by some people as the source of their migraine. When this happens, the patient can restrict their diet. But sometimes it is not easy to pinpoint the cause of the migraine. It is always recommended that the patient eat a diet rich in fresh and natural foods. It is important to use simple cooking methods (steaming, boiling, baking, sauteeing) to help limit salt, meat, and alcoholic or carbonated beverages, very cold foods or spicy foods. It is also important to eat foods rich in vitamin B (whole grain cereals, brewer's yeast), to improve function of your nervous system.

> **Attention to Intestinal Function**
> If the waste from digestion is not passed at least once a day, it can stay in the intestine and generate toxic substances that get into the blood and cause migraines. In cases of constipation, it is sometimes recommended to follow a vegetarian diet for 15 days, eating mostly fruits and vegetables. This will help improve regularity and eliminate toxins.

MANUAL THERAPIES

In other cases, migraines can be caused by bad posture, injuries, or stress that can affect the musculoskeletal system and provoke mechanical disorders that cause migraines. This is where manual therapies like chiropractic or osteopathy can help. A chiropractor searches for the source of the patient's pain in the spine, looking for possible dysfunction that could affect the part of the nervous system that controls the function of the blood vessels in the head, provoking pain. To this capacity, through what are called "chiropractic adjustments" done with the hands, with the help of a special stretcher and simple apparatus, the doctor can re-establish proper communication within the nervous system.

Osteopathy understands migraines to be a consequence of a reflex disorder (due to hormonal, digestive, or tensional causes) that causes an abrupt change in the pressure of the blood circuits in the skull, and that affects the most important arterial roads in the skull—carotid or vertebral arteries. The treatment in this case consists of performing deep mobilizations (if in the viscera), gentle massages (in the head and neck), and also direct maneuvers (if working on the spine), once the diagnosis has been made.

PHYTOTHERAPY

The best remedies that use phytotherapy to fight headaches are the following:

- **Feverfew** (*Tanacetum parthenium*)

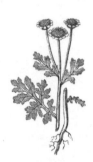

This antimigraine plant is excellent for prevention of premenstrual migraines. Take two cups a day during the week before your period or 10 drops of tincture three times a day. You can also take an infusion that is mixed from equal parts rosemary, lemon balm, and feverfew (a teaspoon of this mixture per cup of water) taken twice a day, best in the morning, or create a

Feverfew

compress with infusion of feverfew (two tablespoons per half-liter of water) and apply to the head, where you feel the most pain.

- **Marjoram** (*Oregano majorana*)

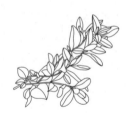

Marjoram is another plant that can help treat migraines. Taken in an infusion (one teaspoon per cup of water three times a day), a tincture (50 drops three times a day), powders, and essential oils for external use.

Marjoram

- **Verbena** (*Verbena officinalis*)

Known for its sedative and antispasmodic effects, verbena is an ideal plant to treat migraines and mild headaches linked to the menstrual cycle, tachycardias, and rheumatic and muscular pain. To prepare a poultice to treat migraines, mix equal parts verbena with linseed flour and fenugreek. Boil until dissolved in milk, stirring occasionally. When the mixture forms a thick paste, spread it on a gauze pad and cover with a piece of cotton to apply to your head where the migraine is. Also you can inhale the steam from the hot verbena decoction.

AROMATHERAPY

Mint (*Menta x piperita*) has an analgesic effect and is useful for relaxing muscles to help alleviate migraines, especially those from tension or nerves. At the first sign of pain, aromatherapy can be applied with a few drops of essential oil (diluted in almond oil) while gently massaging your temples. Do this for about 15 minutes until the pain has passed.

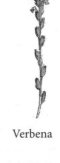

Verbena

Basil (*Ocimum basilicum*) also calms pain naturally. Apply a few drops of essential oil to a cold damp cloth and place it on your forehead for 10 minutes.

Put These Habits into Practice
- **Exercise:** Moderate physical activity can help regulate sleep and release endorphins (hormones related to feelings of wellbeing). For example, walking for half an hour at a brisk pace, swimming two or three times a week, or playing soccer are good ways to prevent and alleviate migraines.
- **Rest:** Sleeping well and without interruptions helps prevent the development of migraines. To do this, maintain a set sleep schedule, finishing dinner no later than two hours before going to bed, and spend some time relaxing before going to sleep (read, listen to music.). Mix a few drops of mint essential oils with three of rosemary, three of basil or lemon, and use on a heater or on your pillow to help sleep.

- **Relaxation:** Stress is one of the main causes of migraines; it is recommended to control situations that may produce stress. There are many ways to manage your stress levels. One is to practice simple relaxation techniques, like a yoga pose or meditation. Bridge pose can be very useful. For this pose, lie flat with your knees bent. Press your arms into the floor along your sides and raise your torso, keeping your head and shoulders against the floor. Breathe slowly and deeply for three minutes (about 10–20 breaths), keeping your body in this triangle. To finish, inhale and hold it for 12 seconds, then relax back to lying on the floor.
- **Auto-massage:** An auto head massage is a good option for managing stress and tension. Place your fingertips on your scalp and press, making gentle circles on your whole head. Work from front to back.
- **Digital Pressure:** Using your fingers to press on certain points (digital pressure) can alleviate pain and relax yourself. Press hard on the fleshy area between your thumb and index finger. You can use your thumb and index finger of the other hand to pinch it firmly. Apply this pressure for 3 minutes, breathing slowly and deeply. Another key point is the base of the skull. Place the middle fingers of each hand there and press from the center out. While maintaining this pressure, exhale and bring your head up slightly. Do this for three minutes.
- **Hydrotherapy:** Perform alternating foot baths. To do this, submerge your feet in a bowl of hot water for three minutes, and then for one minute in a bowl of cold water. Repeat this three times. This helps promote circulation to the head and extremities, relieving pain.

ABDOMINAL PAIN

Abdominal pain is very common, affecting 25–30 percent of the population. Most people have experienced abdominal pain at some point in their life. Luckily, it does not frequently indicate the existence of a serious illness. Pain intensity does not always reflect the seriousness of the illness that causes it. Sharp abdominal pain can be caused by mild illnesses like gas or gastroenteritis, while another light pain can present in more serious illnesses like colon cancer or appendicitis.

There are many organs in the abdomen, and abdominal pain can come from any of these: organs related to digestion (stomach, esophagus, large and small intestine, liver, gallbladder, and pancreas); the aorta (which passes through the abdomen); the appendix; the kidneys, and the spleen. But the pain can also come from another area (referred pain), like the chest or pelvic area.

If the pain is localized (affecting one area of the abdomen) it is probably indicative of a problem in one of the organs, like the appendix, gallbladder, or stomach (like an ulcer).

Colic pain is due to torsion, obstruction or spasms in the smooth muscle that forms the various abdominal viscera. This pain is characterized as being episodic, that is to say it comes in waves, beginning and ending suddenly with frequency and intensity. Kidney and gallbladder stones are common causes of this type of abdominal pain.

The most worrying symptoms are pain that happens frequently, lasts more than 24 hours, or is accompanied by a fever.

As to the possible causes of abdominal pain we find: appendicitis (inflammation of the appendix), intestinal obstruction, cholecystitis (inflammation of the gallbladder) with or without stones, chronic constipation, aortic aneurism, diverticulitis, food allergy or poisoning, epidemic viral gastroenteritis), heartburn, indigestion or gastroesophageal reflux, irritable bowel syndrome, kidney stones, ulcers, pancreatitis, urinary tract infections, menstrual pain.

DIET

When experiencing stomach pain, it is important to abstain from drinking alcohol or coffee, and smoking. Tobacco is a great enemy of a healthy stomach and can provoke harmful effects that assist in the development of and the prevention of healing most gastric illnesses: ulcers, gastritis, cancer, and dyspepsia. At the gastric level, tobacco increases the secretion of acid, reduces the secretion of bicarbonate, mucus and prostaglandins, as well as decreases the flow of gastric mucus.

Spicy and fatty foods will also worsen symptoms over time.

PHYTOTHERAPY

Some medicinal plants can work wonders in the case of stomach pain. Here are some examples:

- **Ginger** (*Zingiber officinale*)
Commonly used in cooking, ginger is an ideal medicinal plant to fight indigestion and its consequences which include nausea, diarrhea, or gas. It is advised to eat lots of ginger when suffering from indigestion.

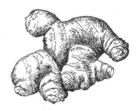

Ginger

> 🍃 *Infusion for colic:* Prepare one tablespoon of ginger root in a cup of water, boil for 3–5 minutes, and take one cup three times a day.

- **Chamomile** (*Matricaria chamomilla*)

Chamomile is a digestive plant with anti-in-flammatory qualities. It is considered to be an excellent remedy to help alleviate indigestion that accompanies stomach pain and gastrointestinal spasms, and a good natural solution against colic. Likewise, it helps to curb diarrhea, alleviate nausea, and prevent vomiting.

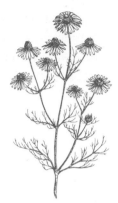

Chamomile

Make a digestive tisane by boiling six to eight chamomile flowers per cup of water for a few minutes. Drain and let rest for ten minutes. It is best to drink it hot, just after eating, to help aid in digestion and prevent pain.

For Babies

Colic is common in four-month-old babies: inconsolable crying that lasts two or three hours where the baby is restless, red, and pushing and pulling its legs continuously. Although it is difficult for the parents, the baby is healthy but having digestive problems. To alleviate this, the baby should be held, rocked, and have its stomach rubbed in circular motions. To help calm the baby, you can also give them chamomile, a gentle and beneficial plant. It is a good idea to make an infusion and give the baby small doses: two small cups a day after meals.

Also with the help of chamomile, in the case of colicky babies, you can cradle them so their head rests in the crook of your elbow and your hand reaches to their diaper. The pressure on their stomach in this position can help alleviate their gas. You can also gently massage their abdomen or perform this exercise: lay the baby down face up and bend his legs up against his abdomen gently to help alleviate the spasm and eliminate gases.

- **Anise** (*Pimpinella anisum*)

This remedy is very effective to reduce the formation of gases and help with their expulsion, because of its carminative effects. This, together with its powers to reduce gastrointestinal spasms, has helped it become a very good resource to help alleviate symptoms of digestive problems like gas and intestinal spasms. It can also help with food poisoning.

If that were not enough, it is also a good antiseptic and expectorant, for treating nonproductive cough, bronchitis, and pharyngitis. It is most commonly used dried, ready to make infusions (one teaspoon per cup of water). Essential oil (0.10 ml a day, distributed in three doses) is another common use. It forms part of infusions to help improve digestion, and also part of some for alleviating colic and other digestive disorders in small children. It is important to note that this plant is not recommended for those who are pregnant or breastfeeding. It is not advised to use the essential oil with children younger than six, or with people diagnosed with epilepsy, or to exceed the daily recommended dose.

> &. *Carminative infusion:* Add half a teaspoon to a cup of boiling water. Let rest 10 minutes and strain. One cup of this infusion, after meals, will help avoid gas and intestinal spasms.
>
> &. *Digestive tisane:* Mix equal parts anise, fennel, and lemon balm. From this mix, add one teaspoon to a cup and add boiling water. Let rest 10 minutes and strain. Take three cups a day, one after each meal.

- **Fennel** (*Foeniculum vulgare*)

Although it smells like anise, fennel is a different plant. Nevertheless, it shares similar digestive benefits. In fact, it is considered an infallible remedy to apply to stomach pain and fights many digestive problems. It is gentle but effective, and has a good flavor which makes it appealing to children with stomach problems and helps stimulate their appetite. Make a carminative tisane by combining one tablespoon of crushed fennel seeds with boiling water. Drink this hot drink after meals. It also helps with morning sickness.

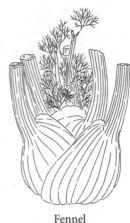

Fennel

SORE THROAT

The throat is a tube that carries food to the esophagus and air to the trachea and larynx. Its technical name is "pharynx". Their conditions are a common cause of pain and can be caused by infections (pharyngitis or viral or bacterial tonsillitis), the passing of stomach content back to the esophagus (gastroesophageal reflux), or serious situations like cancer (the least common). Most causes of throat pain are minor and disappear quickly.

NATURAL REMEDIES

The most effective remedies for throat pain are the following:

- **Oatmeal:** Gargling warm water with oats has a calming, anti-inflammatory effect. It is recommended to do this frequently all day when your throat is sore. Boil two ounces ground oats with one liter water for twenty minutes. Strain and transfer to another container.

- **Garlic:** Garlic is known for its disinfectant properties and it is recommended to be taken raw (most effective), grated (in soups or stews), or cooked in water to make a broth.

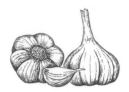

Garlic

- **Tea Tree Oil:** Combine 4 or 5 drops of tea tree oil in a glass of water and gargle with this three times a day (no more) until symptoms are gone.

- **Mallow** (*Malva sylvestris*): This plant has become known as a very effective natural remedy to calm throat pain or bronchitis; it reduces mucus, tonsillitis, and respiratory conditions, and helps fight against the flu. It is most effective in syrup form to help fight colds and flu. You can take up to three teaspoons

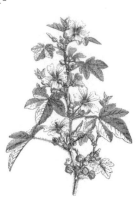

Mallow

a day. An infusion (three small cups a day on an empty stomach) is better in the case of constipation.

PREMENSTRUAL SYNDROME (PMS)

The female reproductive organs (uterus, ovaries, vagina, vulva) are a common source of pain. Sometimes it is difficult to tell exactly where the pain is coming from because these organs are so close to the digestive organs.

There are many different causes, involving different diseases such as dysmenorrhea (pain during menstruation), infections, ectopic pregnancy, ovarian tumors, or endometriosis.

There are many conventional drugs that can be prescribed for premenstrual syndrome (PMS). For example, when the symptoms are bloating, weight gain or sore breasts, nonsteroidal anti-inflammatories (NSAIDs) and diuretics are often prescribed. When menstrual cycles cause intense and incapacitating pain, hormonal treatment is recommended through the use of oral contraceptives. If anxiety, change in character, or depressive states are intense, allopathic medicine can also be prescribed in the form of anxiolytics or antidepressants.

Nevertheless, pharmacological treatments have many side effects, and both short and long-term contraindications, so it is often better for the patient's health and wellbeing to first try a natural treatment. Natural medicine is based on a holistic focus, and looks to not only alleviate symptoms, but also bring balance to the patient's body and mind. Below we will review some of the most effective natural treatments.

Miracle Medicines to Treat PMS

In the last decade, conventional medicine has produced drugs that relieve many symptoms of premenstrual syndrome. Among these, there is one that is the most effective. It uses gonadotropin-releasing hormone (GnRH). This hormone inhibits menstruation and provokes temporary menopause. This drug has little effect on depression as a symptom of PMS.

HEALTHY DIET

A balanced diet should be rich in fruits, vegetables, whole grains and legumes, low in saturated animal fats, and made up of four or five smaller meals eaten over the course of the day. This type of diet can alleviate and diminish premenstrual symptoms. It is also important to get enough vitamin B6, vitamin E, magnesium, calcium, and essential fatty acids.

- **Vitamin B6 or Pyridoxine**

Vitamin B6 or Pyridoxine reduces estrogen levels and increases progesterone. This helps relieve anxiety, irritability, insomnia and depression. It also helps reduce breast tenderness. It is important to follow a diet rich in this vitamin during the week before your period. It is most commonly found in lean red meats, fish, eggs, chicken, and certain fruits including bananas and nuts.

- **Calcium and Magnesium**

Magnesium deficiency can produce generalized pain and decreased pain threshold for menstrual pain. Magnesium can be found in nuts, whole grains, leafy greens, and bananas. Dairy is a good source for calcium, as well as cruciferous vegetables like cauliflower and broccoli, and small fish with their bones, like sardines.

- **Vitamin E**

Studies have shown that vitamin E contributes to a significant decrease in headaches, fatigue, depression, and insomnia. The main sources of this nutrient are wheat germ, olive oil, dry fruits, and whole grains.

- **Essential Fatty Acids**

These should be eaten during the second half of the menstrual cycle to alleviate breast tenderness, headaches, and cramps. Seed oils (sunflower, corn, etc.), olive oil, blue fish, and evening primrose oil are all recommended to help relieve PMS symptoms.

It is also important to drink at least one and a half liters of water a day to help avoid fluid retention. Certain beverages and foods should be avoided during PMS:

- Coffee, tea, and soda all contain stimulants that can increase sensitivity in the breasts, and also potentiate anxiety and irritability.

- Chocolate, sugar, fats (cake, candy, donuts, etc.), alcohol, red meat (and veal, pork and lamb), salt, and other high sodium foods.
- It is important to limit sodium because it contributes to fluid retention, and provokes swelling and tenderness in the breasts. Use herbs and lemon to season your food instead.

PHYTOTHERAPY

Phytotherapy offers a wide range of possibilities to prevent and fight PMS through natural and effective methods without side effects. Medicinal plants are easy to keep and prepare, but it is always important to consult a professional before taking any. Vitex, feverfew, evening primrose oil, wild yam, and passionflower are the most useful for alleviate symptoms of PMS.

- **Vitex** (*Vitex agnus-castus*)

The flowers and fruits from this plant are used for the treatment of PMS symptoms. They help create balance between estrogen and progestogen, to reduce estrogen. It also acts as a mild sedative.

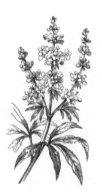

It is found in the form of capsules, and the dosage is indicated by the manufacturer. It is important to keep in mind that this remedy is incompatible with other medications containing estrogen, progestogen, or stimulation of ovulation, for the risk of hyperstimulation. In cases of gestation, its use is contraindicated.

Vitex (also known as Chaste)

- **Feverfew** (*Tanacetum parthenium*)

The tops of this plant are used, due to their analgesic and anti-inflammatory qualities. Feverfew has been used traditionally in the treatment of migraines, arthralgia, amenorrhea, oligomenorrhea, and premenstrual syndrome.

Two cups a day (one every 12 hours) of an infusion or decoction can help mitigate the symptoms of PMS. Its use is contraindicated in cases of hypersensitivity to feverfew or other species in this family and should not be taken when pregnant or lactating.

- **Primrose** (*Oenothera biennis*)

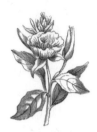

The seeds from this plant produce an oil that is very rich in unsaturated fatty acids; above all linoleic and linolenic acid that helps women relieve the symptoms of menopause. For treating PMS, it is recommended to take this oil in capsules (2–4 grams a day) during the second week of the menstrual cycle.

Primrose

- **Wild Yam** (*Dioscorea villosa*)

The root of this plant is very useful to mitigate the symptoms associated with premenstrual syndrome due to its anti-inflammatory and antispasmodic effects. It helps relieve breast tenderness, muscle pain, pelvic pain, and lumbago. It also calms cramps and alleviates some menopausal disorders like headache, joint pain, and vaginal dryness. It is usually taken in capsules (the dose is indicated by the manufacturer), but you can also find the plant dried and ground to prepare a decoction (two cups a day).

- **Passionflower** (*Passiflora incarnata*)

This is one of the best remedies to diminish nervousness and anxiety, and to prevent insomnia. It acts as a sedative, calming the nerves and relaxing the muscles. It is helpful in stressful situations caused by personal or work problems, and to alleviate the pain of psychosomatic illnesses. It also reduces nervous excitability related to menopause and PMS and has an antispasmodic effect. It is frequently found in form of capsules or tablets, alone or combined with other plants. The appropriate dose is indicated by the manufacturer. It can also be found dried and ground to make infusions (one teaspoon per cup of water), in fluid extract (2 ml every 8 hours), in a tincture (0.5–2 ml every 8 hours). It is commonly used in syrups and other preparations to create a sedative. To calm anxiety, take up to three cups a day (one every eight hours), of the tisane, but do not take in conjunction with sedative drugs because it can have a very strong effect. It should not be used when pregnant or breastfeeding.

PHYSICAL EXERCISE

Together with proper diet and medicinal plants, physical exercise is another useful resource to mitigate the symptoms of PMS. It is well known that it is a fundamental part of a healthy life, but it is also demonstrated that among female athletes, there is a lower incidence of discomfort from these symptoms. Regular exercise can help ease the symptoms of PMS. It is ideal to exercise daily. A half-hour walk at a moderate pace can help improve blood circulation and help decrease headaches and irritability, and also helps improve mood and energy levels. It also has a positive effect on fluid retention. Aside from walking, other sports that help include swimming, biking, jogging, or dancing.

Nevertheless, although a little exercise is good to alleviate symptoms of PMS, too much exertion can result in what is called "athletic amenorrhea." This is when intense and prolonged physical activity causes missed periods. It also influences psychological pressure and stress that can be seen in high level athletes, creating restricted diets.

YOGA

Yoga deserves a special mention. The main goal of this technique is to find balance and harmony between the body and mind. It is proven that people who practice yoga consistently are not only healthy in body but also in mind. There are many different branches of yoga but Hatha Yoga is most suited to relieving premenstrual pain, and it is also very widely taught. If you have never practiced yoga before, it is important to find a studio that will teach you the correct poses and breathing. After the first classes, you should try to practice every day at home for about 10–30 minutes, without rushing. After a few weeks, you should be able to see results from practicing, and the half hour of yoga can become one of the best parts of the day. Here are some exercises that can be done in your home:

- **The Slide:** Lying face up with knees bent, raise the pelvis while tightening the buttocks. Lift it as high as possible, without lifting your shoulders from the ground. Slowly lower back down, focusing on letting each vertebra touch the ground. Hold for 10 seconds when you feel the back and pelvis touch the ground. Do two sets of 10. Afterwards, in the same position but without lifting your back from the floor, move your pelvis in a circle, clockwise and then counterclockwise to help relax the abdominal zone.
- **The Chair:** Stand up and grab the sides of the back of a chair. Bend your knees until they are at the same position as the seat. Hold for a few seconds and return to standing position. Repeat 10 times.

QIGONG

Like yoga, qigong (also known as chi-kung) is a millenary discipline from Asia. It is based on a combination of low-intensity techniques and exercises that help maintain the natural balance between the body and the mind. The exercise is combined with breathing, mental concentration, and physical movement to help increase vital energy, maintain health, and treat illnesses. Studies have been done that show that practicing qigong during the menstrual cycle can help alleviate many symptoms of PMS.

STRESS RELIEF

Every day it is more evident that women suffer from more severe PMS during stressful situations (problems at home or at work, school exams, moving, etc.), rather than when they are more relaxed. It is important to try to avoid stressful situations, both at home and at work, in the days leading up to your period, and try to stay calm. Yoga, breathing exercises, meditation, and other relaxation techniques can help relieve tensions. Reading a good book, listening to music, or taking a walk can be very useful but there are other methods you can do at home to help relieve stress.

- For example, if you have a partner, this could be the perfect moment for them to show off their massage skills.
- Rest is key during these days. You should sleep enough for the body to use its energy for hormonal changes.
- Don't forget to go outside and get some sun. Natural light is a nutrient that the body needs, and to affect the retina, through the hypothalamus and pineal gland, influences the endocrine system. It also influences energy levels, which is why depression can increase during the autumn and winter.
- Share your feelings with your family and friends. This can help you to unburden your problems and feel more relaxed. It is also important to enjoy yourself. Remember that laughing can help calm the nervous system and diminish stress, even if it is difficult to laugh when you are anxious.
- You should also allow yourself some moments of solitude and rest during your premenstrual time, and take a break from your daily duties. It is important to assume that our body needs to rest, and taking time out from your busy life can let you think about, listen to, and reconcile with your body.

AROMATHERAPY

Aromatherapy is based on the use of essential oils to achieve emotional and physical wellness, so that in situations like PMS, in which physical and mental discomfort is so generalized, this therapy can provide subtle, effective, and pleasurable solutions.

- **To reduce fluid retention:** The essential oils from geranium, hyssop, lavender, lemon balm, ylang-ylang, and marjoram can be very useful. A hot bath with five drops of essence of geranium, for example, and another five drops of rose, not only produces a nice smell but also helps alleviate the problem. Another method is a massage, with a combination of 50 ml of a base oil (almond, for example), five drops of marjoram, five drops of ylang-ylang, and five drops of lavender or rose.

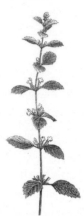

Lemon Balm

- **To calm nervousness and irritability:** The most helpful essential oils are benzoin, bergamot, chamomile, cedar, jasmine, geranium, lavender, marjoram, rose, and ylang-ylang. Baths, aspiration of the essences, and relaxing massages are the best methods to use these oils with. A formula that you can try is the following: 3 ml of bergamot, 3 of lavender, and 2 of rose. To use this formula in a massage, add 50 ml of an oil base (for example, almond), and if you would like to take a bath, add 10 drops to the bath water.

- **When you feel sad or have low energy:** Some essential oils can help mitigate negative thoughts and feelings. These include basil, camphor, orange blossom, bergamot, salvia, incense, ylang-ylang, geranium, jasmine, orange, and rose. The best, in this case, is to use these essences in the bath, or air fresheners. For example, you can combine 6 drops of the mixture with 2 ml of sage and 2 of rose in an incense burner.

HOMEOPATHY

Homeopathy is a recourse to treat and prevent PMS. Even though it is recommended to see a homeopath to prescribe a personalized treatment, the following remedies can help start to alleviate some predominant symptoms of this disorder:

- **For pelvic or abdominal pain:** *Actae racemosa*, *Chamomilla*, or *Belladona*.
- **For nervousness:** *Ignatia*, *Ambra grisea*, *Natrum muriaticum*, or *Platina*.
- **For vascular disorders:** *Lachesis*, *Pulsatilla*, or sulfur.
- **For swollen breasts***: *Laccaninum*, *Bryonia*, or *Phytolacca*.

Remember that it is important to keep the remedies in the receptacle they came in, in a cool, dry place out of the light. It is important to consult a doctor or homeopath if you are taking any other medications. Do not mix these with water as they are already diluted.

REFLEXOLOGY

Conducted regularly as preventative treatment, reflexology can diminish the intensity of menstrual pain. One example is a massage to the buttocks. Standing, place both hands below the buttocks so that the hands and fingers cover the entire buttocks. Perform a massage that works the muscles for a prolonged period of time. It is also useful to massage the feet, where you can find the zones related to the ovaries, lymphatics in the groin, and the pelvic area.

MENSTRUAL PAIN/DYSMENORRHEA

Dysmenorrhea or menstrual pain is defined as abdominal or pelvic pain that appears before or during menstruation. It is considered a serious gynecological problem common in young women (between 25–60% are affected) and is the cause of many absences from work and school. It also causes many women to self-medicate with pain killers.

Dysmenorrhea may occur by itself or accompanied by other symptoms such as nausea and vomiting, fatigue, diarrhea, nervousness, lumbago, dizziness, and headaches. This dysfunction is a syndrome that can harm the physical and psychological state of women who suffer from this periodically.

There are two forms of dysmenorrhea: primary and secondary. Primary is an acute or spasmodic pain in the lower abdomen. In this case, it begins between 24 and 48 hours before the start of the patient's period, and disappears gradually until the end of the first day. It usually occurs in women between the ages of seventeen and twenty-five, and is less common in older women, or women who have had children. Secondary dysmenorrhea manifests as a more steady and deep pain. This dysfunction can begin a week before menstruation and can improve or worsen during the week; it can also persist throughout the entire cycle. It is more common in women older than thirty years old, especially among those who have had children. In the case of secondary dysmenorrhea, it can be a symptom of an underlying illness for which the patient should see a doctor.

The principal cause of menstrual pain is related to the release and increase of the concentration of prostaglandins (chemical substances that play an important role in different processes in our body) due to the disintegration of the endometrium.

To alleviate menstrual pain with conventional medicine, we return to the use of nonsteroidal anti-inflammatories which, even though they have an analgesic effect due to notably decreasing the formation of prostaglandins in the endometrium, they are not exempt from side effects and contraindications.

We recommend certain natural treatments that can be beneficial.

DIET

To begin, the same as for PMS, it is important to watch your diet, giving priority to foods rich in polyunsaturated fatty acids like seed-based oils, olive oil, fish, and whole grains. If the contribution of essential fatty acids was not enough, you can take a supplement in capsule form of primrose oil that we have already discussed in relation to PMS. It has also been demonstrated pain can be relieved through the elimination of coffee, alcohol, simple sugars, and saturated fats, and getting high doses of zinc and magnesium (in whole grains, leafy greens, and legumes) and in vitamin B6.

Drinking plenty of water is also recommended to help with the elimination of liquids, and helping with kidney function. Drinking lots of water can also help relieve constipation which can aggravate premenstrual pelvic pressure. Also eat lots of vegetable fiber found in vegetables, whole grains and fresh fruit.

ACUPUNCTURE AND MOXIBUSTION

These two techniques can be applied to help relieve dysmenorrhea and do not only help alleviate pain, but they also help regulate the menstrual cycle and the function of the genital organs. During menstruation, acupuncture can immediately alleviate the spasmodic uterine contractions that cause a sharp pain.

ACUPRESSURE

Another effective method to fight pain that has no side effects is acupressure. It focuses on certain points and lines on the hands that correspond to different parts of the body. The pressure is made with the thumb and index finger. When you have found the right spot, take your thumb and index finger tip and begin to rub the spot with circular movements, pushing the muscular base or bone with a velocity of about twice per second.

HEAT APPLICATION

Heat applied directly to the belly is especially useful, using either a hot water bottle or an electric heat blanket. This produces a relaxing effect in the musculature that helps alleviate cramps and relieves pain. You can also try clay poultices or warm wet cloths. This relaxes the abdominal muscles.

AROMATHERAPY

This discipline uses essential oils such as cajeput, cypress, juniper, chamomile, marjoram, mint and rosemary, that either alone or combined, help alleviate menstrual pain. For example, you can give yourself a massage on the lower abdomen for the 10 days leading up to your period using the following formula: to 50 ml of a base oil, add 10 drops of cajeput, 10 drops of chamomile, and 5 drops of mint.

SHIATSU

This therapeutic art works the body following the meridians and points from traditional chinese medicine, stimulating the different systems in the body and mobilizing the joints. It promotes the fluid movement of vital energy (Chi) to increase the body's ability to cure itself. To do this, you use pressure from your thumbs, knees, hands, elbows, and feet, along the energy lines in the body and the zones that are needed to release this energy. It is useful in helping relieve menstrual pain. Its role, then, is to channel the extra energy in some parts of the body and move them to where the energy is lacking, looking for a balanced dynamic in the body.

AUTO-MASSAGE

Massaging the muscles in the inner thighs can help relieve the accumulated tension caused by menstrual pain. Open and flex your legs so that the bottoms of your feet almost touch. Create a smooth friction with the palm of your hand moving it from your groin to your knees. It is important to perform this movement in open circles. This helps to unblock the area and relieve pain. You can also use a relaxing oil made from the following formula: 10 drops of marjoram, 10 drops of ylang-ylang, and 10 drops of lavender mixed with 50 ml of almond oil (base oil).

ACCEPT AND RELAX

Your emotional state can influence the menstrual cycle. Dysmenorrhea can be provoked by too much stress or physical tension affecting the pelvic zone. It can also create an aversion to sex or a psychological rejection of the feminine condition. Try to begin to respect your own body.

PHYTOTHERAPY

Phytotherapy offers different remedies to fight this type of pain.

- **Vitex** (*Vitex agnus-castus*)

The use of the flowers and fruits of this plant is common in the treatment of menstrual pain. Its contribution to the alleviation of these pains is due to its ability to modify the balance between estrogen and progestogen.

It is used in the form of capsules and the dosage is indicated by the manufacturer. Nevertheless, before using it, note that it is incompatible with other medicines containing estrogen, progestogen or for stimulating ovulation, because of risk of hyperstimulation. Also do not use if pregnant.

- **Feverfew** (*Tanacetum parthenium*)

The tops of this plant are used, and have analgesic and anti-inflammatory qualities. Because of this, feverfew is used in the treatment of amenorrhea, oligomenorrhea, and premenstrual syndrome, and also in the treatment of migraines and arthralgia (joint pain).

Take two cups a day (every 12 hours) of an infusion or decoction to help mitigate the symptoms of PMS. Do not forget that its use is contraindicated in the case of hypersensitivity to feverfew or other species of the family, or in the case of pregnancy or breastfeeding.

> 🌿 **Combined infusions:** Mix equal parts of the tops of the flowers and fruits from feverfew, salvia, and white hawthorn, adding 1 tablespoon to a cup of boiling water. Strain and let sit 10 minutes. It is ideal to take this every morning when you wake up (on an empty stomach) while the pain goes on.

- **Wild Yam** (*Dioscorea villosa*)

The root of this plant has anti-inflammatory and antispasmodic effects, and is very useful to mitigate the symptoms associated with PMS like breast tenderness, muscle pain, cramps, and lumbago. It also relieves other symptoms of menopause like headache, joint pain, and vaginal dryness. Take it capsules (the dosage is indicated by the manufacturer), and it is also found dried and ground to make a decoction (two cups a day).

- **Passionflower** (*Passiflora incarnata*)

This is one of the best remedies for decreasing nervousness and anxiety and preventing insomnia. Its sedative effect calms nerves and relaxes the muscles. It is very good in stressful situations at home or at work, and can relieve pain from psychosomatic illnesses. It also reduces nervous excitability related to menopause and PMS. Its antispasmodic effect is very useful in avoiding muscle spasm, like intestinal spasms and muscle cramps.

Passionflower

It is most commonly found in the form of capsules, alone or with other sedative plants. The dosage is indicated by the manufacturer. It can also be found dried and ground to make infusions (one teaspoon per cup) in fluid extract (2 ml every 8 hours), and in tinctures (0.5–2 ml every 8 hours). It is often found in syrups and other preparations for sedatives. To calm the nerves and anxiety, take up to three cups a day (every 8 hours) of a tisane, but remember that you should not take this along with pharmaceutical sedatives because it can increase the effect too much. Its use is contraindicated during pregnancy and breastfeeding.

- **Marigold** (*Calendula officinalis*)

This plant with yellow flowers is a useful remedy for menstrual pain, due to its anti-inflammatory and antispasmodic powers. Prepare an infusion by boiling 1 tablespoon of marigold flowers per cup of water for 3 minutes. Take one a day, before meals, and starting 15 days before your period.

Marigold

- **Wormwood** (*Artemisia vulgaris*)

This herbal remedy has been used for its effects on the female reproductive system. It helps regulate the menstrual cycle, calm menstrual pains, and can help in cases of amenorrhea. You can find it dried and ground, ready to prepare infusions. It is recommended that in addition to consuming 3 cups of the tisane a day, you should also prepare hot baths with a few sprigs of the flowers added. If you exceed the recommended dose or take for more than 10 days in a row, wormwood can cause undesirable effects to the nervous system.

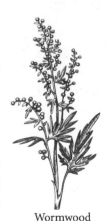

Wormwood

- **Basil** (*Ocimum basilicum*)

Basil has antispasmodic properties, which can reduce menstrual pain. It helps facilitate periods, calm digestive issues due to nervousness, and increases the production of milk in lactating mothers. Basil is a toning plant, which can be taken to mitigate drowsiness and nervous exhaustion. Take as an infusion (1 teaspoon per cup of water, up to 3 times a day) and its use is contraindicated in pregnancy and breastfeeding.

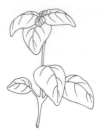

Basil

BREAST TENDERNESS

It is common that after ovulation, breasts become more dense and sensitive as an effect of the hormones produced in the breast tissue in the second half of the cycle. They will feel uncomfortable and tender, for between 2 and 15 days before your period. This pain is known as "mastodynia" and is inoffensive and rarely related to tumors. In the case that it is, it is usually benign and cystic.

In order to relieve this discomfort it is important during these days to use a suitable bra that isn't too tight, and to eat foods rich in vitamin A (eggs, carrots, apricots, cauliflowers) and vitamin E (whole grains, seed oils, and olive oil), and this should reduce discomfort. It is also important to limit consumption of salt and stimulants like coffee, chocolate, or soda. It is also good to have physiotherapeutic massages or hydrotherapy.

Along with pain, it is also normal that nodules or lumps may appear in the breasts during your cycle. Many of these are cysts filled with liquid that grow towards the end of the cycle. If a lump does not disappear after your cycle, see your gynecologist. In young women, breasts are more fibrous and you can feel many nodules in them that disappear completely after the period. It is important to perform a self-examination of your breasts every month; this way you will be more familiar with your breasts and know if there are any changes.

PHYTOTHERAPY

Evening primrose is a remedy that phytotherapy offers to help this kind of pain.

- **Evening primrose** (*Oenothera biennis*)

The seeds from this plant make an oil rich in unsaturated fatty acids (above all, linoleic and linolenic). These components cause good results that are obtained with the use of this remedy in the treatment of different skin problems. Dermatologists are not the only ones interested in its applications, but it also has a great effect in fighting cyclic breast pain. In this case, it is found in capsules (2–4 grams a day) and can be administered during the second week of the menstrual cycle.

ORAL PAIN

TMJ syndrome (temporomandibular joint) refers to a disorder that provokes problems opening and/or closing your mouth, or difficulty with function in the jaw. There are many causes, like strong pressure from chewing, unconsciously clenching your teeth, etc. This damages the teeth and provokes acute or chronic inflammation in the temporomandibular joint that can produce lots of pain in the muscles of the jaw, face, head, back, and neck.

There are many factors that can exercise excessive pressure in the temporomandibular joint, provoking this syndrome, such as: accidental trauma to the teeth, a change in the bite from recent dental treatment that can move the position of the jaw, pressing the teeth (bruxism), or a repetitive movement of the jaw (chewing gum or biting your nails). The principal symptoms of TMJ are: frequent headaches, often when you wake up; difficulty chewing, biting or swallowing; pain in the neck, shoulders or back; pain in the face (sometimes confused with sinusitis); pain in the temporomandibular joint, sound or feeling of rattling in this joint, and pain in the ear.

Often, these symptoms can be alleviated with health education about the understanding of the movement of these joints that can be avoided, and the employment of a brace for when you are sleeping. In certain people that have more complicated problems it may be necessary to try a surgical approach through arthroscopy.

RELAXATION THERAPIES

Relaxation therapies like visualization or meditation can be very useful, since stress is the principal cause of bruxism which causes TMJ.

In fibromyalgia patients, TMJ can cause severe pain in the jaw, face, and neck, and can contribute to headaches. The standard solution is a protective dental appliance (made from plastic or acrylic) from a dentist, created to fit the bite of the patient; the patient wears this at night to relieve pain in the jaw and stress in the temporomandibular joint, keeping the teeth from pressing against each other. To alleviate the muscular pain you can apply a hot, wet towel to the face. There are various treatments, some more conservative while some are aggressive and invasive. In either case, the diagnosis and the therapy should be determined by a dentist who specializes in this disorder.

TOOTHACHES

Maintaining your oral health is not just for appearances. It is imperative to your health. Aside from playing a primary role in helping with swallowing, breathing, and articulation of the tongue, the mouth is capable of expressing a thousand and one feelings. It is important to keep it healthy. Proper hygiene, diet, and some fundamental cautions are not only important for taking care of your mouth but also for your general health. The mouth is the entryway to our bodies, an ecosystem that is home to millions of bacteria, and any harmful substances in the mouth can affect our whole body.

Despite all this, the mouth is often neglected: only a third of Spaniards have been to the dentist in the past year, and 90 percent of those people went because they were experiencing pain, as opposed to just going for their annual check-up. Most people brush their teeth, but many do it wrong, without flossing, only using mouthwash as a treatment, not a prevention. Proof of this is that 90 percent of the population has cavities, and 70 percent has gingivitis.

PLAQUE
To understand what produces dental problems, we need to discuss plaque: a white film that adheres to the tooth, made of numerous bacteria, some of which are harmless, but others have the potential to become sugar acid. It is precisely this acid adhering to the enamel that provokes decalcification in the teeth or creates cavities, which grow from the interior and can cause loss of part of the tooth. Cavities have some symptoms that make them easy to identify: presence of small holes that catch food, pain from hot or cold stimuli. Periodontal disease (or that of the gums) is more difficult to detect in its early stages when it is affecting the bone and gum that holds the tooth. Its principal cause is plaque and tartar (calcified plaque) that forms deposits in the gums. The first stage is the appearance of gingivitis, an irritation, the symptoms of which are pain, blood, and bad breath. If you do not remedy it, it will worsen, affecting the bone, the gums will bleed and begin to lose flesh, and bags where more plaque is deposited begin to

appear. Cavities and periodontal illness are the most common oral diseases and they cause many others, like infections, phlegm, and bad breath.

DAILY HYGIENE

Hygiene is key to enjoying a healthy mouth. It needs to be thorough in order to create healthy saliva as well. The teeth and saliva execute the first steps of digestion, and saliva is also the key to preserving the teeth. It stabilizes the mouth's pH, keeping acids balanced, and it helps prevent plaque, which in turn will help prevent cavities and the destruction of the teeth. And if this were not enough, it contains elements like calcium and fluorine, which help remineralize the teeth and conserve their enamel. The salivary glands produce almost a liter every day, but at night they make less, since the teeth are not being used as much. During the day, it is important to make more to help rinse away food to keep the teeth healthy. "Healthy teeth and gums minimize health problems," says Dr. Jaume Ibarrola, a bioenergetic dentist. Formation of plaque in a healthy mouth, with good gums (without caps or crowns), will be less damaging than if there are already problems.

BRUSHING

"Correct brushing makes up 90% of good oral hygiene, and 95% of the work is done by the brush." With this affirmation, Dr. Ibarrola puts the emphasis on an uncommon method: a dry brush absorbs much more plaque. "Also, by not having that immediate feeling of freshness from the toothpaste, you will brush longer and more consciously," he says. To go along with this, it is advised that you use an interproximal brush or dental floss, to get into the spaces between the teeth. You should then rinse with an essential oil like lemon, myrrh, and cypress. As for mouthwashes and toothpastes, it is best to use natural ones, without fluoride, which despite being a mineral that strengthens teeth, an excess of this can cause damage and be toxic to the body. Ratania, clay, sage, and tea tree oil are effective ingredients present in many of these. It is important to clean your teeth after every meal, even if you can't brush your teeth during the day. You can eat an apple or some sugar free gum to stimulate the secretion of saliva and reduce the development of bacteria.

DENTAL ENEMIES

Refined sugar and starch contribute greatly to the formation of most cavities. They are found in candy and sweets, and in combination have a terrible effect on our teeth. They increase the production of acids that dissolve enamel. The key to maintaining healthy teeth is not to eliminate these foods, but to know when to eat them. Sugars eaten with meals are less dangerous than when they are eaten alone, as eating a meal stimulates salivation and helps reconstruct the enamel. The most dangerous is to snack on products rich in refined sugars (chocolate, candies, cookies, pastries), or foods that have added sugars (precooked foods, prepared sauces, etc), as their cariogenic effect is the same. The frequent consumption of sugar can also contribute to the development of cavities; ingesting these sugars can disrupt the pH of the plaque without leaving it enough time to rebalance. It is crucial to decrease the time the sweet foods is in contact with the enamel, so foods that are chewy or sticky like caramels or honey should be avoided. It is also recommended to suck on them instead of chewing them. Another important recommendation is to use a straw to drink soda or other sugary drinks to avoid direct contact with the teeth.

GOOD FOODS

In addition to avoiding sugar, it is necessary to chew foods well in order to increase secretion of saliva which allows for a quick restabilization of pH levels in the mouth. This, together with the cleaning effects of saliva, helps to easily eliminate any food or sugar left in the mouth. It is beneficial to eat more fruits and raw vegetables that you need to chew.

A healthy and balanced diet can help reinforce the immune system so it can defend itself against infection in the oral cavity. This includes foods rich in calcium (milk, vegetables, dry fruit), phosphorous (cheese, sunflower seeds, almonds, sardines), and fluoride (fish, seafood, tea), and ones that are basic to help preserve the teeth and gums like vitamin D (dairy, eggs), vitamin A (dairy, eggs, fruits and vegetables), that reinforce the enamel; and vitamin C (citrus, peppers, kiwi, strawberries) to prevent illnesses in the gums. Citrus fruits, even though they help make saliva and contain high levels of vitamin C, also contain aggressive acids that severely damage enamel (especially lemons). It is recommended that you do not bite them, but that you drink their juice or rinse with water after eating them.

GENETICS AND MORE

The color of your teeth is determined by genetics, as well as the quality of your gums. But there is no doubt that the caution that we take with caring for our oral hygiene can also influence this aspect of our teeth: "Despite a bad genetic foundation, good hygiene can work wonders," explains Ibarrola. Yellowing of the teeth can also be caused by tobacco and lots of coffee, and abrasive pastes can damage teeth and gums. But besides this unsightly effect and bad breath, tobacco also causes the gums to receive less oxygen and blood, which can weaken them and diminish their resistance to bacterial plaque. If the gums do not bleed, even though they are diseased, it will be harder to diagnose the problem. Alcohol has a similar effect on the gums, as it dries up the mucus and provokes the loss of cells in the tissue that forms the gums, making it easier for bacteria in the plaque to cause damage.

SPECIAL ATTENTION

You need to begin cleaning children's teeth as soon as their first ones come out. It is important to approach this moment with consideration and teach children about oral hygiene from the start. A soft brush with only water will be sufficient at the beginning, until the child is two years old. In elderly people who have suffered a decrease in the production of saliva, it is also necessary to take extra care of their mouth. Certain medicines like tranquilizers, antidepressants, antihistamines, and others that produce dryness in the mouth, can increase the risk of cavities and periodontitis. Women also need to take special care of their mouths during pregnancy. Hormonal changes and the blood flow through the body can cause the gums to become inflamed or infected, and there is also a greater risk of getting cavities. This can affect the dental health of the baby.

Allies of the Mouth

Certain foods and medicinal herbs are recommended to help maintain dental health.

- **Raw Vegetables**: Chewing carrots, apples or celery helps clean the teeth, prevents tartar, and maintains strong gums.
- **Dairy**: Dairy products are a good source of calcium and phosphorus, which help mineralize the teeth. Manchego and gruyere cheeses also reduce acid that forms after meals and impedes the formation of plaque, preventing cavities.
- **Sugar-free Gum**: Chewing sugar-free gum helps facilitate salivation, which prevents cavities.
- **Vegetable Oils**: Include moderate amounts of vegetable oils in your diet, especially olive or sunflower. These oils

help prevent cavities and form a protective barrier on the surface of the teeth, making them less susceptible to be attacked by bacteria.

- **Sage**: Sage is a medicinal plant with strong disinfectant and anti-inflammatory qualities. Adding two drops of sage essential oil to a glass of water to use as a mouth rinse is helpful for inflamed gums and oral ulcers.
- **Tea Tree Oil**: This plant is healing, antiseptic, and antibacterial. You can apply it directly or use in a rinse one to three times a day, using two drops of essential oil to help protect the gums and prevent tartar build up.
- **Clove Oil**: Essential oil from cloves has anesthetic and calming qualities and is helpful in relieving toothaches while you wait for the dentist. Apply three or four drops on a cotton ball to the affected area.
- **Propolis**: Bee propolis is a natural antibiotic that inhibits the growth of bacteria that cause cavities. It can be taken in the form of a candy, tablets, or syrup and is often found in some toothpastes and natural mouthwashes.

PHYTOTHERAPY

Phytotherapy offers different remedies for this type of pain.

- **Sage** (*Salvia officinalis*)

Sores and wounds inside the mouth, weak and bleeding gums, bad toothaches, and throat irritations are all problems that can be relieved with sage due to its astringent, antiseptic, and anti-inflammatory qualities.

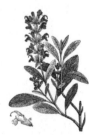

Sage

One good remedy is made by heating two teaspoons of sage leaves in water, removing them from the water once it is boiling, and letting it sit for 10 minutes. Gargle for 15 minutes with the hot infusion. This helps increase the mucus in the mouth and throat to help avoid inflammation.

- **Eyebright** (*Euphrasia officinalis*)

This plant has antiseptic, anti-inflammatory, and astringent qualities and is especially effective against conjunctivitis. It is a classic remedy to alleviate conjunctivitis, blepharitis (inflammation of the eyelid), and eye pain. It is often used in poultices to help relieve styes, and as treatment for eyestrain and other problems with vision related to muscles and nerves. It can also be used to wash rheumy eyes which can help control secretions, reduce inflammation and congestion of conjunctivitis. It can also be gargled to be used against coughs and hoarseness. It is most commonly found dried and ground, ready to be used in infusions (2–3 g per cup of water) or in decoctions. It is also possible to find them in homeopathic eye drops to help take care of eyes, as they are very comfortable and totally harmless.

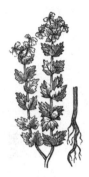

Eyebright

This plant has no side effects or contraindications.

- **Bistort** (*Polygonum bistorta*)

Though it is not well known, this plant is one of the strongest natural painkillers around. It has the capacity to eliminate pain and is ideal for treating mouth sores, bleeding gums, throat irritations, skin wounds, etc.

For a mouthwash to help your gums: prepare a decoction by boiling a half-liter of water with the bistort root, mastic, greater plantain, sage, horsetail, and myrrh in equal parts, about 10 g of each ingredient. After straining, let it sit until it is cool enough to handle, and use as a mouthwash to alleviate pain from mouth sores and inflamed gums.

- **Tea tree oil** (*Melaleuca alternifolia*)

This plant has antiseptic healing qualities. It can be directly applied or in the form of a mouthwash one to three times a day using drops of essential oil each time to protect the gums and prevent tartar.

- **Essential oil of cloves** (*Eugenia caryophyllata*)

This is very useful to help relieve pain while you are waiting to see the dentist due to its anesthetic and calming qualities. Apply three or four drops with a cotton ball to the affected area.

- **Bee propolis**

A natural antibiotic that inhibits the development of cavity-causing bacteria. This can be taken in the form of a lozenge, tablet, or syrup, but also as part of toothpastes and natural mouthwashes.

- **Oregano** (*Origanum vulgare*)

Oregano is a powerful natural anti-inflammatory painkiller that is ideal for alleviating toothaches and earaches. It also reduces joint inflammation. Apply a few drops of essential oil to the affected area and massage two or three times a day.

For toothaches, boil two tablespoons of oregano and poppy with two cloves for five minutes and let rest for another ten. Rinse with this mixture several times a day.

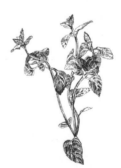

- **Peppermint** (*Mentha x piperita*)

Known for its digestive benefits, peppermint is a plant that can also be very useful

Peppermint

for relieving headaches and toothaches, other oral problems, and muscle and joint pain. Boil 10 grams of peppermint leaves in water to make an infusion that when gargled will help relieve toothaches. This same infusion is ideal as a digestive after a meal.

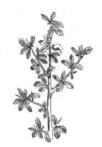

Myrrh

- **Myrrh** (*Commiphora molmol*)
Gargle with a tincture of myrrh dissolved in water.

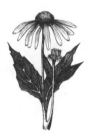

- **Echinacea** (*Echinacea*)
While waiting for a dental appointment, it is recommended that you take 20 drops of a tincture of Echinacea every 4 hours to help prevent major infections, as Echinacea is a plant that stimulates the body's defenses and helps avoid the propagation of infectious microorganisms in the teeth

Echinacea

and gums. You can take the drops alone, or diluted in water, though it is most effective when applied to the damaged area.

HOMEOPATHY FOR TOOTHACHES
Here are several homeopathic remedies for alleviating toothaches:

- **Mercurius:** This is the most commonly prescribed for a toothache, especially if it worsens at night and you are in a humid climate. It is also prescribed for inflamed gums.
- **Chamomile:** This is perfect for toothaches that affect the entire row of teeth, and also radiates to the ears. It is recommended when the pain is worse after eating or drinking something hot.
- **Coffea:** Recommended for very serious toothaches that impede chewing, drinking hot beverages, and when you only find relief when in contact with cold water.

- **Greater plantain:** This is a very effective resource for pain that is worsening and extends to the entire area.
- **Silicea:** Silicea is used for treating dental roots and fistulas. It can alleviate extreme pain that can disrupt sleep.
- **Calcium Fluoride:** This is useful to treat toothaches caused by cavities. It also helps those who suffer from loss of enamel.

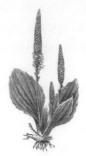

Greater Plantain

PAIN DURING PREGNANCY AND CHILDBIRTH

During pregnancy, many hormonal, metabolic, and anatomical changes occur that can cause different kinds of pain. For example, lower back pain is common, as the back has to support more weight in the abdominal area.

Regarding childbirth, it is well known that uterine contractions cause lots of pain during this process.

During the immediate postpartum period, women also experience genital and breast pain.

Pregnancy and the period after birth is a stage in the life of a woman that can be very painful. In the following lines, we will summarize the most common pains.

BACK PAIN

Back pain is produced by changes in posture that happen when the body adapts to the weight gain or the positioning of the weight and is a very common issue for pregnant women. There are other causes that can explain it: hormones produced during pregnancy soften the ligaments in the pelvis, stretching them to make room for the baby. These pains occur most commonly in those who suffer from cramps during their menstrual cycle. Here are some recommendations for treating this kind of pain:

- Take a relaxing bath with a few drops of lavender essential oil added to the tub.
- Massages with essential oils are very effective. For example, use 100ml of almond oil, 20 drops of essential oil from juniper, chamomile, and lavender. If it is summer, try cryotherapy: make an ice compress and apply it to where you are experiencing pain.
- Pay attention to your posture and try to make sure it is correct to avoid extra tension on the spine.
- Take advantage of the benefits of water, and take a bath or go swimming whenever you can.

MASSAGE

In general, massages during pregnancy are very safe and satisfying, but they are not suitable during every stage. Normally, the second and third trimesters are the best stages to begin prenatal massage. Ideally it is done once a week when you are between three and six months pregnant, and increasing the frequency to twice a week during the last trimester. The body is adjusting to the physical and hormonal changes. In all forms, it is always best to consult a specialist about massages during this time. Among the benefits we find that massages help with the following:

- Alleviate pain and soreness in muscles like cramps, muscular tension, and stiffness.
- Alleviate back pain and reduce fluid retention.
- Help relax the patient physically and emotionally. This is beneficial to both the mother and the baby.

- Stimulate the circulatory system, which oxygenates and nourishes the cells. This process is beneficial to both the mother and the baby.
- Improve the elasticity and tone of the body, which reduces the appearance of stretch marks and varicose veins.
- Help eliminate anxiety and nervousness that sometimes accompanies pregnancy.

HOW TO NATURALLY ALLEVIATE PAIN DURING CHILDBIRTH

It is important to fight the pain in a way that helps the mother relax, as tension can hinder the birthing process. There are natural methods, and others to help fight the pain, like epidural painkillers. Here are some natural remedies:

- **Physical and Emotional Support:** It is most important to surround the mother with confident people in a comfortable environment.
- **Water**: Take a shower or bath in warm water. Not only is this pleasant, but it also helps relieve pain. Some birth centers have special pools for mothers to relax in during the dilation process. There are portable pools in case you are giving birth at home.
- **Heating and Cooling:** Heat stimulates blood flow and alleviates pain. Apply a heating pad to the lower back. If you prefer the cold, use an ice pack or cold cloth to painful areas.
- **Rhythmic Movements:** Go for a walk to stimulate circulation, energy flow, and oxygen.
- **Homeopathy:** Homeopathy can help not only treat pain but also your attitude if you are scared or anxious.
- **TENS (Transcutaneous Electrical Nerve Stimulation):** This method consists of applying electrical impulses through

patches on the skin to alleviate pain, usually in the lower back and the abdomen. It is harmless and effective, but expensive.

After childbirth, the breasts begin to produce milk, in a natural process that helps feed the baby in the upcoming months. Before they make the milk, the breasts first secrete colostrum, an intense yellow liquid with a high amount of proteins and antibodies.

CONGESTION

The increase in milk occurs within a few days of giving birth. If it takes longer, it can be painful. The breasts can feel very full, like they are going to explode. In this case, if the baby cannot drink all the milk, you can extract the milk from your breasts and keep it to give the baby later. It lasts up to three months in the freezer. You will need sterilized containers or hermetically sealed bags. If you simply want to alleviate the feeling of congestion, you can massage the breast and apply heat until the milk comes out. It is also helpful to direct the stream of hot water from the shower towards your chest, moving it in circular motions until the milk comes out easier. Another solution is to let the baby drink more frequently. Other methods are:

- Try to breastfeed often. Sometimes engorgement is due to skipping a feeding, or when the baby begins to sleep more during the night. It can be useful to maintain nighttime feedings.
- Correctly empty the breasts at every feeding.
- Apply heat to the breasts after every feeding, to help alleviate the symptoms.
- Apply crushed parsley leaves to the breasts.
- Place a bag of ice on the engorged breast between feedings to relieve discomfort.

- If the baby will not latch onto the breast, manually extract the milk so he can try again.
- Be observant, and try to use correct techniques and positions for breastfeeding.

CRACKS IN THE NIPPLE

Sometimes breastfeeding can cause a lot of pain. Often, the nipples develop cracks. Every time the baby latches to the nipple, the mother will feel like she is being stabbed with a thousand needles. Sometimes they can begin to bleed. This is where rubber nipples come in handy. They are a latex protector (like a teat or a bottle) that are placed over the nipple and allow for the baby to suckle without making direct contact. The baby may have to suck harder to get the milk, but after a few days the cracks should heal and the baby can continue feeding as usual without the rubber nipple. Once they heal, they do not come back. Other than the artificial protector, you can use:

- Special creams for the nipples, especially lanolin, after feeding.
- Another effective method is to massage the nipples with a few drops of milk after feeding. It is a good lubricant and stops the proliferation of bacterias, and alleviates cracks.
- Marigold (calendula) cream calms and heals painful cracked nipples and is harmless to the baby.
- Caraway, anise, and fennel, when taken as an infusion, can help stimulate the production of milk.

MASTITIS

This is an inflammation of the breast that is sometimes infectious. It is a disorder that produces fever, general discomfort, and inflammation. The breast is red, hot, and painful. It usually affects one side.

It is important to be treated by a doctor, and ensure good posture for the baby during feeding. It is necessary not to suppress the lactation, and it is also important to extract the milk when you have mastitis. The best way to do this is to continue having the baby feeding. There is no reason a woman with mastitis should stop lactating, and if there is a stop in the lactation, there is probably an abscess.

POST-PARTUM YOGA

For those of us who enjoy exercise, yoga can be a good alternative. In fact, experts in this field agree that if practiced regularly during pregnancy, it can help with problems of weight gain, back pain, and fluid retention. It is also helpful during birth to help diminish the pain of contractions. Another advantage of this technique is that it helps with emotional stability and once the baby is born, it reduces the possibility of postpartum depression.

FIBROMYALGIA

Although it is not new, there is a lot that remains unknown about this illness, which is becoming more and more frequent. It affects mostly women between twenty and fifty years old, and it is not an inflammatory process. Nevertheless, it is an illness characterized by prolonged pain in the whole body, with hypersensitivity and rigidity in muscles, joints, and soft tissues. This pain travels from one part of the body to the other and its intensity fluctuates: sometimes it diminishes during the day and increases at night, even though it is more frequently present all of the time.

This pain is classified among rheumatic chronic illnesses, and although it is not serious, its multiple symptoms can be associated with a high degree of suffering and incapacitation if not treated, which is not easy to do as it is difficult to diagnose. This is because its symptoms are very generalized and indeterminate. While there is no test to diagnose fibromyalgia, rheumatological institutions have developed some standards to be able to diagnose it. According to these parameters, they consider a person to be suffering from this illness if they have been in pain for at least three months, and suffering from pain and sensitivity in at least eleven of the eighteen trigger points. These points are at the base of the neck, the length of the vertebral column, at the hips and elbow and behind the knees and shoulders.

Aside from pain, symptoms include fatigue, stiffness in the morning, sleep problems, tension headaches, difficulty swallowing, recurrent abdominal pain, diarrhea, numbness or trembling of the extremities, depression and anxiety.

There is still no known therapy to treat this chronic affliction, but the objective of treatment can be focused on alleviating the symptoms.

The treatments are directed to reduce pain and improve the quality of sleep. Deep sleep is fundamental to the various function of the human body (like repairing tissues, regulation of neurotransmitters, hormones, and immunological substances) and it is believed that sleep disturbances in fibromyalgia patients are an important factor in maintaining the symptoms of the illness. Low doses of serotonin are often prescribed, as it is a neurotransmitter that helps modulate sleep, pain, and immune response). A large variety of analgesics are also prescribed, the most common of which is paracetamol.

The majority of these patients, however, need other auxiliary treatments like physiotherapy, gentle exercise, heat, massages, and other prescribed techniques.

For this reason, the conventional natural treatment can necessitate the combination of various therapies, exercise and advice necessary to adopt the best lifestyle. That is to say, the key to treating this illness is a holistic focus on oneself. Nevertheless, though the treatment should be individualized, there are several methods that are very useful to each person that suffers from this illness.

WAYS TO ADOPT A HEALTHY LIFESTYLE

- Diet should be healthy and balanced and include a wide range of fresh fruits and vegetables. It is necessary to diminish the consumption of saturated fats (meat, sausage, etc.) and avoid caffeine and other stimulating drinks (coffee, tea).
- Fish oil, combinations of magnesium and malic acid, or vitamins can help treat this illness.
- Improve your physical state with exercise. Studies have demonstrated that aerobic exercise is most effective in alleviating the symptoms of this illness. The best way to begin a physical training program is with low impact like walking and swimming. Start slowly to help tone sore muscles. Aerobic exercises of high impact and weightlifting might increase pain.
- Maintain correct posture and do not overwork yourself carrying or lifting heavy weights that you are not prepared to lift.
- Control your weight as obesity and weight gain can aggravate symptoms.
- Lots of rest is necessary to treat fibromyalgia.
- Be careful of your psychological state and maintain good motivation and outlook on life. Also, protect yourself from stress, anxiety, and depression, seeking out psychological help to ensure a balance in mood.

PHYTOTHERAPY

The use of certain medicinal plants is a good natural method to mitigate pain, purify the body, and improve sleep.

- **White willow** (*Salix alba*)

The root of the willow can be used in a decoction (2 teaspoons per cup, every 8 hours), in capsules (the dosage is indicated by the manufacturer), a fluid extract (1 or 2 ml every 8 hours), and as a tincture (between 5 and 8 ml every 8 hours). But remember not to use this if you are allergic to salicylates, or have gastritis, peptic ulcers, asthma, alterations in blood, or to use for children under twelve years old. It is also not recommended if you are pregnant or lactating.

- **Passionflower, valerian, and lime blossom**

Among the best remedies to decrease nervousness, anxiety and fight insomnia, we have passionflower, valerian, and lime blossom, among others. These plants have a sedative effect that helps calm the nerves and relax the muscles. They are good in stressful situations and to alleviate pain from psychosomatic illnesses. They are useful to take in an infusion (one cup every 8 hours), in capsules, or tablets (the dosage is indicated by the manufacturer).

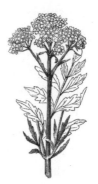

Valerian

- **Birch** (*Betula pendula*)

Purifying plants like birch increase urination and help with the expulsion of uric acid, while decongesting joints. In this case, it is good to take an infusion (1 or 2 teaspoons per cup, twice a day), and it can also be found in capsules or tablets (the dosage is indicated by the manufacturer) and in fluid extract (3–5 ml a day, taken in three doses). It is not recommended for use during pregnancy or

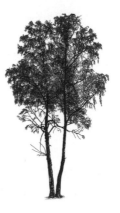

Birch

breastfeeding, and in the case of kidney or cardiac issues, you should consult with a specialist before use.

HOMEOPATHY
Among the most commonly used homeopathic remedies to alleviate symptoms of this pain, we have *Kali phosphoricum, Phosphoricum acidum, Gelsemium, Picricum acidum*, and *Avena sativa*.

OTHER NATURAL REMEDIES

- Hydrotherapy exercise (in a bathtub or pool) can be useful to provide low impact exercise which can relax muscles and eliminate joint pain.
- Exercises for relaxation like yoga, and other relaxation therapies can be very useful and help with total wellbeing.
- Baths or compresses with lavender, chamomile, or juniper oil use aromatherapy to alleviate muscular and joint pain.
- Light massage and chiropractic (preferably in short sessions) are also useful to help with symptoms.

SOPHROLOGY
This therapy was created in 1961 by Professor Alfonso Caycedo and is based on therapeutic experiments and personal investigations carried out in India, Tibet, and Japan. Sophrology helps the whole body as well as the mind. Through positive stimulants in the mind, the intent is to normalize or diminish negative mechanisms responsible for the illness that affects the body.

ENDONASAL THERAPY
This is a technique that improves illnesses related to abnormalities in the sympathetic nervous system like stress, nervousness, sleep disor-

ders, and neurovegetative endocrine disorders. The technique consists of stimulating endonasal nerve endings in the sympathetic system, located in specific points of the nasal passages, with blunt-tipped points that have a form and composition adjusted to the desired effect. You can also use certain essential oils on the tips for a potent and long-lasting effect. This is done over between five and fifteen sessions, once or twice a week, and the effects can last a few months.

BIOFEEDBACK

Evaluating and observing information related to the body's temperature (related to blood circulation in the muscles and tissues), muscle tension (related to electrical activity in the nerves and muscles), the cardiac rhythm, and emotional state.

This relationship between the mental state and physical body is not usually consciously perceived. The work of biofeedback consists in trying to be more conscious. Circulation, muscle tensions, and breathing can be altered in fibromyalgia; biofeedback can help you be more conscious of an activity that needs to be corrected. This way the person affected by the fibromyalgia can gradually regain control of their body's functionality and improve their quality of life. This control is obtained through recognition of normally subliminal signals.

OZONE THERAPY

This consists of the subcutaneous application of ozone at the paravertebral level and above the painful points, followed by a massage to distribute the injected gas. This creates hyperoxygenation in the muscular tissue, reducing pain.

MESOTHERAPY

This therapeutic method from France is well known in Europe, where it has been practiced for more than thirty years. It consists of subcutaneously injecting small quantities of a mix of medicines appropriate for the symptoms. The technique is used in the treatment of muscle and tendon pain characteristic of fibromyalgia. The sessions use a series of injections in the painful zones and sensitive points.

DIET

In recent years, we have seen that a change in diet can help reduce pain and discomfort for fibromyalgia patients.

- Give priority to foods that are grown in the earth. Fruits are full of vitamins, minerals, fiber and sugar. Vegetables are rich in vitamins, fiber and mineral salts. Legumes and vegetables, along with whole grains, are the base of a healthy diet. Rice, corn, bread and pastas are a good source of carbohydrates and vegetable proteins.
- Substitute animal fat for vegetable. Animal based foods increase the possibility of inflammation.
- Avoid processed foods and condiments. Do not cook pre-cooked food.
- Reduce the consumption of sugar. Do not add sugar to foods and pay attention to ingredients, as many products have added sugar. The kinds of sugars that are recommended are those present in fruits, honey, milk, and certain vegetables like carrots and beets.
- Limit salt consumption to avoid edemas. Processed foods are high in sodium, which is not good for your health.
- The ideal drink is water or infusions. Eliminate juices and sodas, as these are high in added sugar.

People with fibromyalgia usually go through a critical period between eleven and sixteen hours long, during which they feel most tired.

When someone is in this state it is best to have a snack and some water to return their energy. It is recommended that people with fibromyalgia drink one or two liters of water a day. Medication can dry out the mouth, and it is good to drink a little water every ten to fifteen minutes. You should not drink alcohol. There is no known cure for fibromyalgia. Nevertheless, just the same as other disorders, it is important to follow a healthy and balanced diet, exercise regularly, and rest enough.

Ranking of Pain According to the International Pain Foundation

- Fibromyalgia
- Lumbago
- Sciatica
- Osteoarthritis

Osteoarthritis pain in the knee is the second most frequent pain in the whole population. It is due to bipedalism because all the weight of the body rests on the knees. The factors that can aggravate this problem are weight gain, spinal alignment, different lengths in the legs, stepping wrong, or limping. These situations alter the vegetative nervous system creating an immunological disorder that can end in destruction of the joint, like an autoimmune disease.

BACK PAIN

Eighty percent of the population has suffered or will suffer from back pain at some point in their life; a number that increases to 90 percent among people older than sixty-five years of age. Back pain, whether lower, dorsal, or cervical, constitutes the second most frequent cause for missing work. Lumbago is the most common chronic pain among humans, because of our posture and walking on two feet. This causes strong pains in the base of the spine, extending to the buttocks and the backs of the legs, which can prevent us from standing up straight. The lumbar zone is most affected by back pain. According to statistics, four and a half Spaniards suffer from lumbago, an illness with is chronic in half its cases. Eighteen percent of women suffer from lumbago, as opposed to 11.3 percent of men. This discomfort is the price humans pay for being bipeds rather than quadrupeds. Some experts say that our species is not evolved enough to support this posture without consequences, as all the body weight rests in two lumbar vertebras, the fourth and the fifth.

Our body is designed for constant movement, flexibility and dynamism. Our lifestyle however, creates large blocks of time during which we are inactive, sitting in the same position. Eighty percent of back pain has a functional origin, i.e., they are not caused by an injury in the vertebral spine, but are caused by a malfunction in the muscles, ligaments and joints. This is usually produced by an overexertion, a disturbance to the ligaments that connects the muscle to the bone, or cramps due to an excess of nervous tension. The first step to preventing back pain is to be attentive to your everyday posture and exercise regularly to strengthen your back.

Why Does My Back Hurt?

- **Carrying Too Much Weight:** If there is too much stress on the musculature, it is easy to develp painful contractures.
- **Too Sedentary:** Decrease in muscle tone due to a sedentary lifestyle causes muscular fatigue and increases pain in the spine.

- **Postural Imbalance:** Deviations in the spinal column (scoliosis, lordosis and cifosis) and static injuries in the feet (flat foot, cavus foot) can provoke misalignment and discomfort in the back.
- **Psychoaffective Disorders:** Increased anxiety and depression can manifest on a physical level and have repercussions to your back health.
- **Climate and Temperature:** Changes in climate, humidity, cold, and wind can cause back pain.

By following these simple preventative measures, you can avoid most back pain:

- **Do not overload your body:** To maintain good posture at home and work, make sure you rest and take a ten-minute break when you need to.
- **Get a good mattress:** It is essential to sleep on a medium-firm mattress, not too soft, and not too hard. Your pillow should support your head and neck, and not let your head rest at an angle.
- **Exercise regularly:** Practicing regular physical activity like swimming, gymnastics, walking, or bicycling can help maintain muscular tone in the spine. This should be combined with a daily regimen for stretching to eliminate tension and rigidity.
- **Maintain your weight:** Avoid weight gain, as extra weight puts strain on your joints and back.
- **Wear comfortable shoes:** Shoes, especially women's shoes, should not be completely flat, or have a heel over 2–3 inches high.
- **Have a positive attitude:** It is important to maintain a good attitude and remain optimistic that the pain will go away.

These habits contribute to reducing the health costs that back pain generates, as doctor's visits can include many diagnostic tests like MRIs, CT scans, or electromyograms.

When the pain begins, specialists recommend rest for the first two days, applying heat to the sore area with a cloth or hot water bottle. Muscle relaxers are often prescribed, with a warning that they may produce drowsiness and should not be taken with alcohol.

Staying in bed for more than two days can be damaging and affect your ability to maintain physical activity to keep the muscles and bones strong. You lose flexibility if you do not exercise, making it more difficult to return to normalcy. Your doctor can recommend specific exercises to perform regularly to help relieve back pain. These include walking, swimming, cycling, or corrective gymnastics.

When Is Surgery Necessary?

Only 10 percent of lumbagos need surgical treatment. Eighty-five percent can be cured with conservative treatment over 2–3 weeks. There is often discordance between symptoms and what is observed in scans (tomography, MRIs), and it is important to be prudent before deciding to operate without having tried several therapies first (physiotherapy, postural work, epidurals) and acquiring a second opinion. Often people continue to experience back pain even after surgery, making surgery a very rare solution.

ELECTROTHERAPY

Electrotherapy employs a series of techniques that are used frequently for treatment of chronic and acute back pain. They apply energy through a certain type of wave to raise the temperature in the deep tissues.

The application of heat with preheated objects or hot water has been demonstrated to be effective to relaxing muscles and for analgesic and anti-inflammatory effects. The problem with this mode of applying heat is that it does not deeply penetrate and does not reach the muscles or tendons situated more than a few centimeters below the skin.

Electrotherapy solves this problem by using different sources of energy, like ultrasounds or short wave, with the end result of being able to apply deep heat, improving the vascularization of tissues and accelerating the healing process.

ULTRASOUNDS

Ultrasounds consist of applying ultrasonic waves to the patient in the form of vibrations, penetrating about 5 centimeters into the soft tissue.

The tissues that absorb most of this energy are the muscular tissue and nervous tissue. When applied in a fixed point, pain can develop from heating the area too much; to avoid this, the apparatus needs to be moved continuously. You can use this without problems with patients who have metal implants (unlike other techniques that use electrotherapy). Ultrasounds can decrease pain and increase mobility. They can also help relax muscles by warming the muscles by a few degrees.

Ultrasounds are used to apply local medicines, like cortisone, local anesthetics or anti-inflammatory creams, instead of injecting these through the skin.

SHORT WAVE

These are electromagnetic waves of high frequency that increase temperature in the tissues. The muscle can heat to temperatures of around 100°F, which will relax the muscle and improve circulation. The treatment usually lasts twenty minutes. Short wave can also accelerate the healing process for wounds and hematomas.

This method should not be used for people who have hemorrhagic illnesses as it may produce hematomas. It should also not be used on parts of the body with metal implants like pates or prosthesis, because it can heat the metal too much and injure the surrounding tissues. It should also not be used with a pacemaker as it may damage it.

TRANSCUTANEOUS ELECTRICAL NERVE STIMULATOR (TENS)

TENS is an effective method of controlling acute or chronic back pain. It consists of a low voltage electrical current applied to the patient.

Some studies have been done that show that the application of TENS decreases pain in 60 percent of patients to whom it is applied.

Electrodes are applied to the skin on the injured zone. The electrical stimulation that the patient receives should not be uncomfortable. The stimulation should be maintained for 30–60 minutes for chronic problems, and up to 2 hours for acute problems.

ELECTROANALGESIA

This method is more difficult to apply than TENS, and is used for treatment of acute back pain. It consists of the application of a low voltage electrical current on the classic acupuncture points for sixty seconds at a time. This can relieve pain in only one session.

BACK SCHOOLS

Back schools developed in the 1960s in Switzerland at Volvo's automobile factories, extending later to the rest of the world. Today there are thousands of back schools operating on every continent. The objective of the back schools is to educate the general population about posture in order to prevent back problems. The people who most regularly attend these schools are those who have had back problems, although anyone is welcome.

EXERCISE: THE IDEAL PREVENTION

A sedentary lifestyle causes loss of strength in your muscles, and causes lots of back pain. It has been proven that people who exercise regularly suffer from less back pain, and can recover from injury faster. Exercise increases bone density, strengthens musculature, helps maintain flexibility, produces endorphins, and reduces stress which can also improve back pain.

Even if you are experiencing discomfort, experts advise that you be as active as possible and practice exercise a little at a time, such as walking or swimming. Swimming is especially recommended to help prevent back pain. It helps because you can move all of your joints and muscles without feeling too much weight on them. This is thanks to the effects of being underwater, where the body only weighs 10 percent of its real weight. The two recommended strokes are the front crawl, and the back stroke. Breaststroke is not advisable because it puts too much stress on the cervicodorsal musculature; the butterfly stroke also provokes detrimental curvature of the lumbar zone. And in cases of lumbago, above all it is necessary to strengthen the back with exercises specific to the abdominal muscles, which support the lumbar zone. Exercises that strengthen muscles through symmetrical movements can help in these cases (swimming, walking, and other aerobic activities).

During pregnancy and labor, the spinal column and the musculoligamentous joints undergo a process of adaptation that can cause discomfort if you do not take preventative measures, like stretching or practicing gentle exercises (like walking).

We should keep in mind that the spine is like an archive of the activities that we have done in our lives. If we have not corrected our bad habits as we age, we will have more and more problems. Tobacco increases the risk of back pain, and blocks the irrigation of the intervertebral disc and causes coughs, which increases pressure in this zone. Smokers' musculature is often in worse state than non-smokers. Personality can also contribute to the pain, if you are anxious or unhappy, this can increase back pain.

POSTURE

The posture that we adopt for most of the day and while we are sleeping will directly affect our back. For example, when we are sitting, the intervertebral disc bears the load of our weight (which can range from 60 and 140 percent of what we carry on foot). Even if you are not in pain, you should develop a daily routine to help maintain our posture to avoid overloading the muscles resulting in discomfort.

According to different scientific studies, learning to pay attention to our posture daily can prevent more than 60 percent of work absences caused by back pain. We are the ones who can help ourselves the most. Here are some guidelines to help develop good posture:

- **Standing**: Shift your weight from one foot to the other every five minutes, and occasionally rest against a wall to take the weight off of the spine. Keep your ears, shoulders, and hips in a straight line, the head lifted, and the stomach contracted.
- **Sitting**: Sit in a chair with a straight back, supporting the lower part of the back. Keep your knees higher than your hips and adjust the seat to make sure your feet touch the floor. Use a foot rest.
- **Driving**: Bring your seat forward to better reach the pedals, and so that your knees and hips form a right angle. Rest a cushion behind your back.

- **At the Computer**: Position yourself so that the screen is at eye level and directly in front of your face. To type, make sure your arms are raised above the table.
- **Watching Television**: It is important to avoid armchairs or sofas that are too low. Make sure your shoulders and back are supported (place a cushion behind your lower back). Lift your feet and rest them on a stool.
- **Sleeping**: Face up, keep your knees bent with a pillow underneath them.

PHYSIOTHERAPY

The goal of this technique is to diminish the most pain, relax the musculatura, improve mobility, and stimulate blood flow.

Exercises are personalized for each patient and each illness, helping adjust the patient's posture to avoid pain, contractures and deformities in the spine; applying techniques like massage therapy, stretching and mobilizing muscles; applying heat through deep thermotherapy (ultrasounds, microwaves, etc.); and with electrotherapy of low and medium frequency, that reduces pain and relaxes contracted muscles.

It is indicated in spinal pain (cervicalgia, dorsalgia, lumbalgia, ciatalgia), scoliosis, arthrosis, osteoporosis, and discal hernias.

CORRECTIVE GYMNASTICS

One type of gymnastics focuses on reteaching morphological alterations in our body. It is preventative and can help patients become more conscious of their correct posture that they should adopt in their daily life. These exercises develop strength and flexibility, and improve balance. It is recommended for people affected by back pain, postural problems, rheumatic illnesses, or who simply want to prevent future problems. Some techniques like Pilates are considered to be corrective gymnastics.

OSTEOPATHY

This technique has gained recognition at an academic level. It considers the body to be one unit and holds that emotional stress, traumatic injuries and incorrect posture can all affect the musculoskeletal system, internal organs, and the function of the body's systems both directly and reflexively.

Osteopaths are dedicated to making adjustments in joints, muscles, soft tissues, and between different organs and body systems. Their work helps reestablish the correct balance between these parts.

Lumbar pain is one of the problems most commonly treated by osteopaths. They apply a series of precise techniques to the damaged area. These manipulations, when done correctly, do not present any risk or side effects for the patient, aside from slight stiffness and fatigue that can appear immediately after an injury.

Lower back pain is a problem that is usually treated by osteopathy. The professional examines the spine to detect the stiff zones and applies a series of techniques with the goal of relaxing these areas.

Most of the time, only one or two sessions are enough to help, but in some cases it can be necessary to employ prolonged treatment over several months. The first consult can last about an hour and the following are not usually more than thirty minutes long. The majority of the professionals spread the sessions over two or three weeks so that the body can assimilate to the changes. The osteopathic treatment can be combined with other psychotherapeutic treatments and the specialist can recommend that the patient perform exercises and techniques for relaxation at home or at work.

GLOBAL POSTURAL REEDUCATION

Global Postural Reeducation (GPR) holds that the body depends on a set of forces between different muscle chains. The appearance of pain in our body can provoke other short-term or long-term problems.

GPR individually analyzes each body to evaluate the postural problems and to correct them through personalized exercises. These distend or strengthen determined muscles in the body.

The principles of GPR are: individuality (it is centered on the study of each patient), causality (the problems and their solution are explained by the action of concrete forces), and globality (the diagnosis and the treatment are based on the idea that the body functions as one unit). It is effective for back pain related to postural problems and deformities in the spinal column like scoliosis, kyphosis, lordosis, and herniated discs. In the case of herniated discs in particular, GPR can help render surgical intervention unnecessary.

CHIROPRACTIC

Chiropractors help with the diagnosis, treatment, and prevention of alterations to the neuro-musculoskeletal system, especially the vertebral column. It treats the effects that these disorders produce (vertebral subluxations) in the nervous system and in health in general.

Chiropractic adjustment is the method of correcting and diminishing vertebral subluxations. This can help reestablish communication in the functions of the nervous system and restore balance and harmony in the body. Many studies support the efficacy of chiropractic in relieving pain caused by back problems (herniated discs, lumbago, sciatica). It also has many other indications in general.

ACUPUNCTURE

This is a basic treatment in traditional Chinese medicine that relates health to the harmony between the complementary energies of yin and yang. Acupuncture treats disorders in the body as imbalances in energy.

The specialist places fine needles along the body in certain points that correspond to internal organs. With this, they can reestablish the flow of vital energy. The session helps the patient relax; it is not painful and does not draw blood.

REFLEXOTHERAPY

This therapeutic massage technique is performed on the feet. It is based on the idea that the whole body is reflected in the feet, and massaging the nerve endings can simulate the different organs in the body.

YOGA

This therapy, among other benefits, is a great option to correct spinal problems and, above all, improve flexibility and posture. This is achieved through breathing, postures (asanas), and relaxation.

MASSAGE

Based in the stimulation of soft tissue and the vital functions of the body through the hands, massage is recommended for back pain originating in contractures and rigidity in the muscles. Massage also helps improve circulation and has a relaxing effect, which help relieve tension and stress, two primary causes of back discomforts. Through massage, the body is manipulated in one form or another depending on the kind of massage employed, and can produce effects in the muscles and circulatory and lymphatic systems. There are several kinds of techniques like full body alignment, Californian massage and energetic massage (like Tibetan, ayurvedic, shiatsu, tuina, and Thai, among others).

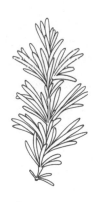

Rosemary

You can also rub the injured area with rosemary alcohol. This can be found in the pharmacy, or prepared with a jar of 96 proof alcohol and three tablespoons of fresh rosemary. Let steep for one week, agitating the jar periodically. Strain the liquid and keep in a dark bottle to keep out light.

HYDROTHERAPY
When you suffer from back pain, it is advisable to take a hot bath to which you have added essential oil of juniper to relax the damaged muscles.

PHYTOTHERAPY
Many plants that we have mentioned for treating rheumatic pain are also useful in treating back pain. We will describe some of the possible remedies.

- **Devil's claw** (*Harpagophytum procumbens*)
This is useful for treating back pain provoked by inflammation in the joints. Mix equal parts 20 g devil's claw root, white willow bark (which contains salicylic acid) and viburnum bark. Boil in 750 ml of water. Strain and let sit for 10 minutes, taking two or three cups daily depending on the intensity of the pain. You should see results after a week of treatment.

> **Sciatica (or sciatic pain)**
> Sciatica is a pain that is felt from the lumbar spine down the back of the thigh and leg, all the way to the toes. It can be caused by damage to the sciatic nerve or the compression of the nerve roots where they exit the spinal cord. Other illnesses could cause similar pain. This pain usually continues or grows when you are in a certain position, coughing,

sneezing, or making another sudden movement. It most often affects men between the ages of twenty and forty.

You are more at risk for sciatica if you have a job that requires considerable physical force, or you have bad posture, or play dangerous and forceful sports. Obesity and a sedentary lifestyle and low muscle tone, osteoporosis, and other illnesses that affect the bones in the spine can all also contribute to sciatic pain. It is necessary to maintain good habits to avoid it, like sleeping in a hard bed with a straight back.

- If you have to lift heavy objects, do so carefully, with correct posture, and holding the object close to the body.
- Do not lift from the waist, but from the knees.
- Try to use correct posture, and do not change position suddenly.
- Exercise to improve muscle tone and lose any excess weight.
- Wear appropriate footwear when performing specific activities, and, if it is necessary, use a back brace in the workplace.

Possible consequences of sciatica are that this pain can restrict activity and if the pain continues with frequency over a long period of time, it can worsen your quality of life. It is necessary to call a doctor if you are feeling pain in your lower back for more than three days in a row, if the episodes are happening frequently, if new symptoms appear, or if there is no improvement during treatment.

Treatment is not complicated and can have good results; however, if you do not eliminate the cause of the pain, it will not ever go away for good. Sometimes surgery is necessary. Depending on the severity of the episode, the doctor can prescribe bedrest, painkillers to alleviate the pain, and immobilize the zone with a brace. Sometimes the doctor will recommend certain exercises to help reduce the pain (sometimes this is more effective than prolonged rest). It is also advisable to get massages from a chiropractor. Surgery can be done in the case of severely herniated discs, tumors, or for prolonged and frequent episodes.

CERVICAL PAIN

One of the most common pains in traumatology is cervical pain. It used to be seen as something specific to certain professions (secretaries, models, staff of an assembly line), but today it is attributed to a sedentary lifestyle, which has extended to all professions that involve working in an office and using a computer.

Over many years it was believed that back pain, and by extension cervical pain, was caused by alterations in the structure of the spine that caused problems. In these last years we have learned that this is not supported by scientific evidence, and thanks to radiographic tests we have learned that those who suffer from these illnesses have demonstrated that the majority of times the pain in the cervical column comes from bad posture and insufficient muscle strength. This generates inflammation and muscular contractures.

Cervical pain can originate from various structures in the neck, such as muscles and nerves, or vertebrae and the cushioning discs between them. It can also come from other areas of the body near the neck, like the shoulders, mandibula, and the upper part of the arms. When the neck is injured, it can be difficult to turn your head side to side, which is called a stiff neck or torticollis. If the pain in the neck involves the nerves (for example, large muscle spasms that involve a nerve, or a displaced disc that presses on a nerve), it can produce numbness, tingling, or weakness in the arms, hands, or other parts of the body.

It is important to pay attention to cervical pain and treat it correctly. Cervical arthrosis can affect the bones. The pain can become chronic and remain despite adequate rest, causing the patient to not be able to move their neck and have difficulties in their daily life, like when driving or doing physical work, diminishing their quality of life.

Approximately 25 percent of men and 35 percent of women have suffered from cervical pain in their lives, and this is just one type of pain among the back problems that affect 80 percent of the population. Among people under sixty years old, back pain in the cervical column more frequently affects women, but after this age the terms are reversed and it is mostly men who suffer from this kind of pain. One of the reasons to explain this is that women have always been more sedentary than men: performing more physical exercise strengthens the cervical area.

Elderly people are a group that also suffers from cervical pain: about 90 percent of this age group is affected. In these cases, the degenerative musculoskeletal process associated with advanced age and coupled with the emergence of diseases such as osteoarthritis is responsible.

A GOOD DIAGNOSIS

The first step in fighting this kind of illness is to see a family doctor, especially if it is the first time that you are experiencing this pain. The doctor will analyze your pain and its possible cause and if necessary, refer you to a specialist: traumatologist, rheumatologist, neurosurgeon, and/or rehabilitation or pain clinics.

If you know you slept in a bad position or injured yourself with a sudden movement, you can take certain measures to alleviate this: apply ice for the first 48–72 hours and then heat (with hot showers or compresses or heating blankets). It is also recommended to perform cervical exercises with slow movements, up and down, side to side, and from ear to ear, to gently stretch the cervical muscles.

If the pain persists, it is necessary to see a doctor. Normally, a study of the statics of the spine will be necessary to conclude if the vertebras are affected and provoke pain, or if it is created by an organic problem.

ADEQUATE TREATMENTS

Treatment of cervical pain depends on the diagnosis. In general, almost every person sees results through rest, medication, immobilization with a collar, physiotherapy, exercise, or, if necessary, a change of job. Treatment varies according to the type of pain: acute (lasts less than fourteen days), subacute (between fourteen and ninety days) or chronic (more than three months). In the first case, the most effective therapy on a pharmacological level are anti-inflammatories, analgesics, and muscle relaxers prescribed by the family doctor or specialist. When the pain is subacute or chronic, the administration of treatment should be individualized through study: normally pharmacological therapies are combined with other techniques. One of these techniques, despite lack of scientific evidence, is neuro reflexotherapy. This consists of the superficial implantation of surgical staples over nerve endings in the skin. They are implanted about 2 mm deep in the affected area, in this case on the cervical or dorsal level (trapeze and interscapular area). These staples have neurological effects that reduce inflammation, pain, and contractures. Some natural therapies can be used. Homeopathy can create long-term treatments (not in specific crises); acupuncture as shock therapy in the moment of crisis can reduce pain; and chiropractic and osteopathy can unblock contractures.

Relaxation exercises like yoga or tai chi are recommended to help with breathing, self-control and relaxation, and improving posture.

PHYTOTHERAPY
Phytotherapy offers an effective remedy for this kind of pain.

- **Viburnum** (*Viburnum*)
Viburnum can be prepared as a lotion that is very useful in the case of neck pain. Prepare a decoction with 30 g of viburnum bark.

Why Does My Neck Hurt?
It used to be that neck pain was associated with aging, but it really is found more frequently in people between thirty-five and sixty-five years of age, ages that coincide with your working life. Tension, anxiety, and bad ergonomics in the environment create this common illness whose prevalence is growing. Cases of cervical pain exist in children: 70 percent of school children under the age of sixteen suffer from this pain, almost always because of an excess of weight in their backpack. Below we explain other common causes of cervical pain.

- **Trauma**: One of the most common causes of cervical pain is whiplash, which affects 25,000 Spaniards a year. This is a neck injury caused by a car accident, contact sports, or from diving into water. It is benign.

- **Stress**: Nervous tension produced by a period of stress and anxiety can provoke a muscular overcharge in the neck.
- **Bad Posture**: Using a computer, sleeping, watching television lying down, carrying heavy bags etc.
- **Pulled Muscle**: Turning the neck quickly and roughly while doing exercise, dancing, or in another moment, can produce muscular tension or distension.
- **Other Causes**: Alterations to the body (herniated discs, fibromyalgia, and arthritis) can cause pain.

IMPROVING POSTURE

Our neck suffers from our habits during the rhythm of life, a summation of tension that we cannot release, which can become chronic. Generally, neck pain is not directly related to injuries, but is related to an imbalance in nervous control of the musculature, which is subjected to repeated contraction, reducing blood and lymph risk. If there is not a specific injury, the neck pain is the result of a sum of tensions that affect the nervous system, from which continual discomforts originate, including partial or total immobility that can limit our capacity to move. If an injury is ruled out, we can look for the true source of the problem and figure out at what point we lost control of our situation. It can also be interesting to think about our emotional and mental attitude and how that can contribute to the growth of tension and pain in the neck. The most common cause of cervical pain is incorrect posture with the head hanging down and rounded shoulders, which not only hurt the muscles that support the head, but also cause the upper part of the chest to tighten, causing breathing problems. As the muscles become gradually tenser around these points, this can cause pain in other tissues. A recommended treatment can be to stretch the muscles that have tensed, deactivating the trigger points and improving posture. Some helpful techniques include: physiotherapy, chiropractic, osteopathy, and muscular massage.

The majority of people pass many hours a day in front of a desk and with their sight focused on a computer screen. This activity can create bad posture where we round our shoulders over and push our head forward. This is usually done unconsciously and it is difficult to correct. It is important to constantly try to correct the muscles in the neck and shoulders.

What Can I Do About Chronic Neck Pain?

First of all, it is important to consult with a professional to find any injuries, and in the case that an injury is ruled out, the most recommended treatments are to find good posture, practice exercises that strengthen muscles, and search for causes that create tension in the neck. It is also effective to perform auto-massage on the affected area and apply clay poultices, because this can reduce stiffness in the neck and shoulders.

Moving the head slowly from side to side while breathing deeply, will help alleviate tension. It is also helpful to shower with hot water. It is advised that you put the back of your neck under the stream of the shower, and move the head in ways that will stretch the muscles. It can help to do this every day, especially at the end of the day.

- Sit on the edge of a seat with your feet firmly planted on the ground (if you are wearing high heels, it is best that you remove them), hips-width apart, and with your toes pointed out.

- Pull your chin a little bit inward and let your arms hang at your sides with your palms facing forward.
- Inhale, and while exhaling, turn your arms clockwise so that your thumbs remain pointing out, and stretch your fingers. At the same time, raise your sternum forward, and arch the lower part of the back. Relax, and repeat this five times.

RELAXATION

Stress, physical as well as mental, is the principal cause of tension in the neck. Practicing the following exercises several times a day can help reduce rigidity, improve mobility in this area, and increase blood circulation in the head.

- **Loosen Up:** Standing, or sitting comfortably with back straight and shoulders relaxed, inhale slowly while lifting your head up. Then, in one continuous movement, exhale and bow the head back down. Repeat 5–10 times, slowly.
- **Stretch:** Put one hand on your head (above the opposite ear). Pull firmly and gently until you feel your neck stretching. Meanwhile, lower the shoulder and relax the arm, and exhale air with each stretch. Do this exercise three times per side.
- **Relax:** Clasp your hands behind your neck and raise your head up. Inhaling deeply, press on the base of the neck with your hands and lift your head back farther while you exhale. Repeat this exercise 3–5 times.
- **Activate Energy:** Place your fingers on the base of the skull, just to the side of the cervical vertebras. Press gently and deeply, without it hurting. Slowly raise your head back while you

exhale. Press in different places to find different muscles. Do this exercise again on the other side.

- **Tone the Neck:** Take a rolled towel and hold it tightly by the ends. Place it behind your neck and pull firmly. Creating resistance, lift the head back and then turn the head from side to side gently against the towel. Do this 10 times, breathing and loosening the neck.

IT'S ALL ABOUT ATTITUDE

- **Optimism:** A positive attitude can help facilitate the treatment to help fight pain and improve results.
- **In Shape:** Physical and mental activity, daily exercise (like walking), and correct posture can improve the quality of life.
- **Have Fun:** Something as simple as relaxing can help relieve pain. In the case that pain is causing you to abandon a fun activity, you should find something to replace it.
- **Look for Help:** Pain can have a heavy psychological impact on the life of the affected person. It is important to find a psychologist. These specialists, through relaxation techniques, can teach people with chronic pain how to improve their situation.

EAR PAIN

Otitis can affect different structures in the ear. It can be otitis externa (also known as "swimmer's ear" due to its prevalence among people who perform aquatic sports), otitis media, or otitis interna.

Otitis externa is most common in the summer. It affects the external auditory canal and develops from bacteria and spores present in water, which alter its acidic pH and favor the nesting of microorganisms susceptible to produce infections. This is common in children.

If water has gotten into their ear after swimming or showering, and has not been removed, try to move their head from side to side. If the feeling of tamponade does not stop, you can get some drops from the pharmacy that contain alcohol which, when it evaporates, absorbs the water and helps the ear dry. It also has an antibacterial and anti-fungal effect. If after everything an infection occurs, it can be treated with a few drops that contain antibiotics and anti-inflammatories which also help rebalance the pH in the external ear.

One of the principal causes of ear infections, especially in the summer, is water. At first, taking a bath may not seem to be very risky, but if liquid enters the ears, it can cause problems. It can cause microorganisms that alter the pH and cause infection to grow.

Infections occur most of all in contaminated water, like rivers and pools. Often, although we have taken the necessary precautions to avoid microorganisms present in water, we can still develop ear infections.

Otitis media is a persistent inflammation of the mucus that covers the middle ear. It produces a liquid exudation that accumulates and remains trapped in the Eustachian tube, which causes pain and hearing problems. The most common causes are: suffering ear infections many times, the presence of an infectious obstruction in the Eustachian tube, a mechanical obstruction (vegetation), or an allergic obstruction. Some microorganisms can be responsible for this otitis.

In the case of otitis interna, inflammation is produced in the inner ear or labyrinth. Although the cause is unknown, specialists think that it can be derived from untreated otitis media or an infection from the respiratory system.

PHYTOTHERAPY

For otitis, medicinal plants are recommended for us to help fight these problems naturally. On one hand, they present as a resource for our defenses, and on the other hand, they have antiseptic and anti-inflammatory actions. Many kinds of ear pain can be fixed with natural remedies from plants. The anti-inflammatory and antiseptic effects of cloves, mullein, can help relieve these pains. Do not put anything in your ear without the advice of a specialist.

- **Cloves** (*Eugenia caryophyllata*)

Cloves come from a tropical tree related to the eucalyptus. It contains an essential oil, rich in eugenol and caryophyllene, and is considered to have great therapeutic value. Above all, it is known for its powerful antibacterial, antiseptic, and antiviral properties, and on a local level it has been shown to be an effective anti-inflammatory and analgesic.

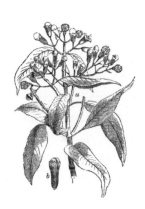

Cloves

Essence of clove (or macerations of clove in olive oil) have been shown to be very useful when applied to earaches in babies and to reduce infection in the auditory canal. Remedies with clove, in fact, are recommended for all types of otitis, as they are good for odontalgia, tonsillitis, mouth sores, and skin ulcerations.

Cloves can be used when cooking to season stews and salads, as spice mixtures, and in making candies and perfumes. It is also a good natural air freshener.

Take orally as an infusion (three cups a day), in drops of essential oil dissolved in oil, or as a powder. Essential oil taken orally should be avoided when pregnant or breastfeeding, and with children under six years old.

- **Mullein** (*Verbascum thapsus*)

The flowers and leaves of mullein are used as an effective natural remedy for all kinds of issues in the respiratory system (which is often the origin of infections) thanks to its balsamic, expectorant, and antitussive qualities.

Mullein oil, obtained from macerating the inflorescences, also have demonstrated to have an anti-inflammatory capacity to palliate ear pain. Its application reduces the formation of fluids in the auditive conducts, facilitates the purification of these fluids, and prevents irritation and inflammation. In the same way, the use of these drops can alleviate burns, superficial wounds, sores, furuncles, and other skin problems.

It is known for diminishing the formation and accumulation of mucus and helping with the expulsion of phlegm from a cough. In this sense, remedies with mullein can be very helpful when treating moderate otitis caused by a cold.

Take as an infusion alone or mixed, up to three cups a day; in a concentrated decoction with a cloth or compress.

- **Satureja** (*Satureja fruticosa*)

This plant is an aromatic bush commonly found in the low mountains of the Mediterranean coast. It contains essential oil, rich in pulegone, flavonoids, and rosmarinic acid, among other active ingredients that create a remarkable antiseptic and antibacterial action.

In external application, white pennyroyal is especially effective to prevent infection in cutaneous wounds, sinusitis, conjunctivitis, blepharitis, and otitis (above all otitis media). A few drops of its infusion, or of its essence, can be used to fight infection in the middle and inner ear: it stops viruses and prevents nausea and acute pain, and in serious cases, loss of balance.

Tisanes, prepared with its freshly picked flowers, has been considered to be a good digestive balsamic. To fight otitis, this Mediterranean plant can be taken as an infusion (two cups a day with food) or in drops (two times a day).

- **Cotton lavender** (*Santolina chamaecyparissus*)

The flowers of cotton lavender share similar therapeutic qualities with chamomiles; they are digestive balms and a good anti-inflammatory and antiseptic remedy. For external use, apply to fight oral infections, blepharitis, conjunctivitis, and otitis. It also contributes to reduce inflammation localized in the middle and external ear and neutralize the bacterial action from the accumulation of sterile fluids in the auditive conducts. If the otitis continues and you are suffering nasal congestion, inhale the fumes from this plant one or two times a day for relief.

The essence, in isotonic solutions is used to clear the nostrils of mucus that blocks the ears. Take an infusion with a few drops, or have three drops three times a day.

HOMEOPATHY

Homeopathy can be very effective when otitis has a component of stress and antibiotics are not working. For acute attacks, you can apply Viburcol, as a suppository every 2–3 hours. If the pain does not stop, 7–8 drops of Traumeel in the auditive conduct along with the suppositories can help. The relief should be quick.

AROMATHERAPY

Essential oils can be helpful to fight earaches.

- **Lavender** (*Lavandula angustifolia*)

Traditionally, to alleviate pain, a few drops of warm olive oil were applied inside the ear, but this risks introducing substances, including plants, that could worsen the infection. It is better to soak a cotton ball in a warm solution of lavender and pat the ear with this. This oil has calming and disinfecting qualities. This can be applied several

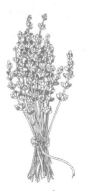

Lavender

times a day, but it is most important to do this before bed and during the night.

HEAT
Apply a heated cloth over the affected ear to produce great relief.

NERVE OR NEUROPATHIC PAIN

This kind of pain is produced by an injury or illness in the somatosensory system. It can occur because a nerve is affected or it is near an affected tissue. It is usually a poorly localized pain that is difficult to describe (cold, hot, a tear, a cramp, needles, weight, etc) and can persist after the apparent cause that produced it has disappeared (for example, a painful scar after a mastectomy, lung removal, or inguinal hernia).

This type of pain, because of its characteristics, persists despite an absence of objective injuries and can be misunderstood or misjudged by family, friends, coworkers, or doctors.

An example of this type of pain is shingles. The fact that it hurts can be what makes a nerve inflamed and cause the outbreak, usually around the ribs. But it can appear in any nerve in the body (eye, face, arm, leg). It is very important to calm the pain before an outbreak to keep our brain from memorizing this pain. This way if we cannot control the pain with medication, it is recommended to find a pain expert who can help find adequate treatment to keep this from becoming a chronic condition. It is difficult to avoid the appearance of postherpetic neuralgia that consists of the persistence of pain over time even after the shingles have healed. This neuralgia is more frequent in older people and people with low immunity.

Diabetes is another possible cause for neurological pain. While many forms of pain may stem from diabetes, the most common is burning pain and numbness in the feet, like a sock. Fortunately, good control of diabetes prevents its appearance, and in case it does develop, good care can delay or prevent its worsening.

Treatment with Drugs

- **Antidepressants:** Antidepressants have been very useful in low doses (without an antidepressive effect) for the treatment of neuropathic pain. They are especially useful to control oppresive, tense and continuous pain. In low doses, they have very few side effects, the most common being drowsiness and dry mouth. The most commonly used is amitriptyline.
- **Antiepileptics:** Antiepileptics are another family of drugs that has been very useful in the treatment of neuropathic pain. Over many years Tegretol (carbamazepine) has been used in the treatment of trigeminal neuralgia. Currently there is a new generation of antiepileptics with fewer side effects and equal efficacy (gabapentin, pregabalin). They are especially useful for controlling intense pain.
- **Lidocaine:** Lidocaine is a drug with different applications as a local anesthetic or for treating cardiac ventricular arrhythmias. Because of its effect in reducing nervous excitability, it is used in the treatment of neuropathic pain via blood.

CANCER PAIN

Eighty percent of advanced and terminal cancer patients suffer from pain. In fact, it is the second symptom that manifests, following asthenia. It can be provoked by the cancer, but also by its treatment (surgery, chemotherapy, radiology), or by other unrelated causes. Persistent pain is usually treated so that the patients often turn to pain units, in which specific treatments are applied.

Cancer pain is very complex. Especially as the pain advances, many different kinds of pain coexist. In pain clinics or pain units in medical centers, they have experience managing the many medications prescribed by oncologists. They also have the capacity to apply techniques that permit an acceptable reduction of pain up through very advanced stages of the illness, while preserving the consciousness and quality of life. It is always convenient to make therapeutic pacts to continue adapting the resources to control pain at the request of the patient and their family. Especially in the more advanced stages of the illness, even though there are only a few remaining weeks in the patient's life, the presence or absence of pain can be very important. Here the doctor can apply techniques like epidural blocks, nerve blocks, or epidural or intrathecal infusions of analgesic medications to improve the patient's life, without pain and with waking consciousness. Evidence exists that good control of pain in the hands of experts can prolong the length and quality of life.

In any form, it is not only useful to visit a pain clinic in the final phase of an illness, but when pain is difficult to control, you should visit the clinic, no matter what stage you are in an illness. It is important to understand the work that is done is a joint service provided with other specialties. The ideal situation is to collaborate with the service of an oncologist. The correct therapies applied will diminish or eliminate pain.

MORPHINE AND OTHER OPIATES

Before we address the question of whether morphine provokes addiction, we should first clear up the terms "dependency," "addiction," and "tolerance." Tolerance implies the necessity of progressively larger doses to obtain the same therapeutic effect. This happens with morphine but does not usually cause problems because there is no ceiling. That is to say, every time you increase the dose, the desired effect increases. Secondly, it also creates a tolerance for the side effects that begin to disappear with the passing of time.

Physical dependency means that if the treatment is suddenly interrupted, the patient can go through what is called "withdrawal," a series of unpleasant symptoms that can be eliminated by resuming treatment or taking a tranquilizer.

Psychological dependency is what is commonly called "addiction." It happens when the use of morphine has a different effect than normal. Among people with chronic cancer pain, versus non-cancer chronic pain, the frequency of developing an addiction is less than .2 percent.

In the case of a patient who needs more morphine, this can be a phenomenon of their own tolerance to morphine, but also the progression of the illness can necessitate a higher dose.

In the same way that pain treatment is begun, the ladder of medications becomes stronger and stronger, but you can go back down the ladder and stop the morphine treatment if the illness is going away and the cause of pain is disappearing.

"I took morphine and now I am very nauseous. Does this mean I should not take opiates?"

The response of different opiates (morphine, methadone, fentanyl, buprenorphine, oxycodone, tramadol, codeine) is individual and depends on the amount and type of receptors that we have in our brains. Because of this, one bad experience in one patient does not mean that another patient will not have success with the same drug.

"*Are there other opiates besides morphine?*" As we have said, there are other drugs, either synthetic or derived from opium, that have properties that interact with the Mu and Kappa receptors. Among these, the most commonly used are fentanyl, buprenorphine, methadone, tramadol, and codeine. Presently, we have options to take these drugs through oral, transcutaneous, orally transmucosal, endovenous, or epidural methods. These methods can have fast, slow, or long-lasting action. They are usually combined with one long-lasting action to help the patient through a pain crisis.

Practical advice about transdermic opiates (DUROGESIC®, TRANSTEC®): It is important to observe the recommendations of the manufacturers. It is necessary to be careful with the skin because the patches they use can cause local irritations. It is also important to keep in mind how quickly the medication passes from the patch to the skin and into your blood depends on the skin's temperature. Because of this, when you have a fever, you run the risk of overdosing if you are not careful.

Medication in a patch does not have a localized effect below the patch, as the medication passes to the blood through the skin and has effects on pain throughout the body.

"*I have rheumatic pain that is not getting better. Should I keep using opiates for cancer pain?*"

Every time it is accepted more that when pain is intense, you must treat it with strong drugs regardless of its origin. There is plenty of experience and publications that support the use of opiates in patients with chronic non-cancer pain without finding complications or incidence of addiction higher than among cancer patients.

POST-SURGICAL PAIN

In the world of pain therapy, controlled analgesic systems can be like the Rolls Royce of treatment for the patient. It is an intravenous infusion or epidural that allows for the continuous administration of medication, but also, that the patient can self-administer when they need extra, without risk of overdose because the system is programmed to avoid this.

The use of PCA systems (Patient Controlled Analgesia) is growing every year. In our center we use these regularly, although with restricted indications due to its high cost.

CHRONIC PELVIC PAIN

According to the Spanish Society of Pain, one of the prime challenges presented in pain clinics is chronic pelvic pain (CPP), produced by illnesses in the structures of the lower abdomen, that are located in the pelvis or the area nearby. The prevalence of these pains is unknown and published studies say the same.

In a high percentage of patients (10–50 percent), the cause of pain remains unidentified after having completed many diagnostic procedures (image studies, laparoscopy, etc). It is necessary to note that an important number of people who suffer from chronic pelvic pain have a history of sexual abuse.

The treatment of pelvic pain is as broad as the pathology capable of producing the pain. The first is intended to identify the cause and treat it in consequence. It is necessary to have a multidisciplinary approach that includes physiotherapy (exercises for the pelvic floor, massage, etc.), pharmacological treatment with medications for neuropathic pain (anticonvulsants, antidepressants) or non-steroidal anti-inflammatories and/or opiates according to the case. Psychological treatment has a certain role, with techniques for relaxation, hypnosis, biofeedback, etc.

When this treatment is not able to help the patient, creating peripheral nerve blocks is the next step (blocking the pudendal nerve), sympathetic system nerve blocks (blocking the hypogastric plexus and the odd ganglion), or including neurostimulation in the sacral roots, has been demonstrated to be effective in select patients with interstitial cystitis.

VULVODYNIA

This name is given to a procession of symptoms among which we find pain in the vagina or vulva, which can also include the anus, and the perineal fascia. This syndrome is related to neuropathic pain and secondary stimulation of the sympathetic nervous system in the area.

The cause of vulvodynia is many times unknown, but it can be related to aggressive procedures in the area (curettage, forceps), scars, infections, dermatological illnesses, problems with the surrounding joints (hips, pelvis), or psychological traumas that produce maintained contracture of the muscles of the pelvic cure, and can cause, among other things, the neuropathy of the pudendal nerve.

It is an entity that is difficult to diagnose, and it is important to go see a specialist who will conduct a fracture history, a complete clinic, and adequate exams.

Treatment is a challenge for the specialist. Even though the pathology is related to neuropathic pain, it can be treated with drugs that have shown effectiveness in calming this kind of pain (anticonvulsants, antidepressants, tramadol). Opiates and anxiolytics are also used (above all those that treat anxiety related to the pathology), with varied results. When drugs fail, interventional techniques can be employed like nerve blocks for the pudendal nerve, or selectively in the sympathetic system (hypogastric, odd ganglion). We should note that psychological support is fundamental in treating vulvodynia. Physiotherapy techniques for relaxing the pelvic floor can help in many cases to diminish the pain brought on by this pathology.

SHOULDER PAIN

Shoulders can hurt when an arthrosis is produced in the joint, the subacromial joint or the supraspinatus ligament, which is injured very frequently when the shoulder is hurt from lifting weight. The pain is confounded sometimes with that from cervicalgia, because it is produced in the neck and sometimes in part of the shoulder.

OSTEOPOROSIS

Osteoporosis at first does not produce pain; because of this it is called the "silent illness." Pain from osteoporosis is produced by fractures, and more concretely, the last dorsal vertebrae crushing together. Osteoporosis occurs mostly in women between sixty and seventy years old. The main cause is the lack of secretion of estrogen that occurs during menopause or early sterilization in a woman. Another cause of osteoporosis is immobilization or treatments with corticoides. The vertebra that usually are crushed are the ones from the ninth to the eleventh.

TENNIS ELBOW (Lateral Epicondylitis)

Tennis elbow is pain in the external part of the elbow caused by continuous microtraumas caused by certain sports like tennis, paddle tennis, or golf. It can also be found in people who catch weight in certain positions: lifting patients or giving your arm habitually to people for support.

This is one of the most common injuries that occurs in your arm. It is an injury that is associated normally with work, playing sports, or practicing another activity that uses a repetitive movement in the arm or wrist. This produces inflammation in the tissues that surround the lateral epicondyle that affect the external muscles of the wrist. Common symptoms are pain and loss of normal function that interfere in daily activities in patients.

PHANTOM LIMB

Pain that presents in patients after having suffered an amputation. The nerves are cut and send erroneous information to the central nervous system (medula and cerebral cortex) that translates to pain from the loss of the limb. Whether lost in an accident, or removed surgically, amputations have great repercussions for those who are affected. There are three main problems:

- **Phantom Sensation:** This is a non-painful sensation that is felt in the amputated part of the body. It occurs in 90 percent of patients within the first few months of the amputation.
- **Phantom Limb Pain:** This is pain that occurs after the amputation with neuropathic symptoms (burning, tingling, electricity). And it is frequently in people who have suffered from

previous pain. It is important to treat quickly because when it becomes chronic it can be very difficult to eradicate.

- **Stump Pain:** This is pain localized to the stump and is related to the presence of a local problem (infection, pneumonia, a badly adjusted prosthesis).

NERVE ENTRAPMENT

This is common in its many forms. One cause of this pain is small nerve roots within scars after an operation. The scar is formed by conjunctive tissue that is called "fibrosis," which can engulf and compress the nerve root, producing pain that is difficult to diagnose because it radiates to other areas. Carpal tunnel syndrome is an example of nerve entrapment.

Bibliography

Aliaga, L. *Conferencia en el Queen Sofia Spanish Institute.* New York, December 19, 2010.

Aliaga, L. *Dolor agudo y postoperatorio.* Barcelona: Caduceo Multimedia, 2005.

Aliaga, L., Baños., J. E., Barutell, C., Molet, J. and Rodríguez de la Serna, A. "Tratamiento del dolor." *Teoría y práctica*, 3rd ed. Barcelona: Publicaciones Permanyer, 2010.

Bell, I. R., Lewis, D. A., Brooks, A. J., Schwartz, G. E., Lewis, S. E., et al. "Improved clinical status in fibrom-yalgia patients treated with individualized homeopathic remedies versus placebo." *Rheumatology*, 2004, 43(5):577–582.

Berna, C. H. "El estado de ánimo deprimido guía el dolor y lo empeora." *Diario Médico*, June 10, 2010: 22.

Bertolini, A., Ferrari, A., Ottani, A., Guerzoni, S., Tacchi, R. y Leone, S. "Paracetamol: New vistas of an old drug." *CNS Drug Reviews*, 2006, 12 (3–4): 250–275.

Bonica, J. J., Loeser, J. D. "History of pain concepts and therapies." In *Bonica's management of pain*, 3rd ed. (Ed. J. D. Loeser). Philadelphia: Lippincont Williams & Wilkins; 2001: 3–16.

Bosch Llonch, F., Bañoz Díez, J. E. "Conceptos generales en algesiología." In *Tratamiento del dolor: Teoría y práctica*, 3rd ed. (Ed. L. Aliaga). Barcelona: Publicaciones Permanyer, 2009: 3–7.

Bosch Llonch, F., Bañoz Díez, J. E. "El dolor a través de la historia." In Tratamiento del dolor: Teoría y práctica, 3rd ed. (Ed. L. Aliaga). Barcelona: Publicaciones Permanyer, 2009: 3–7.

Breivik, H., Collen, B., et al. "Survey of chronic pain in Europe. Prevalence, impact on daily life, and treatment." *European Journal of Pain,* 2006, 10: 287–333.

Busquets, C., Ribera, M. V. "Unidades del dolor." In *Unidades del dolor: Realidad hoy, reto para el futuro* (Eds. C. Busquets, M. V. Ribera). Barcelona: Acadèmia de Ciències Mèdiqus de Catalunya i Balears, 2002: 47–52.

Casals, M., Samper, D. "Epidemiología, prevalencia y calidad de vida del dolor crónico no oncológico." *Revista de la Sociedad Española del Dolor*, 2004, 11: 260–269.

Catalá, E., Reig, E., Aliaga, L., et al. "Prevalence of pain in the Spanish population: telephone survey in 5000 homes." *European Journal of Pain*, 2002, 6: 133–140.

De Barturell, C. "Historia del tratatmiento del dolor." In *Unidades del dolor: Realidad hoy, reto para el futuro* (Eds. C. Busquets, M. V. Ribera). Barcelona: Acadèmia de Ciències Mèdiqus de Catalunya i Balears, 2002: 47–52.

De Silva, V., El-Metwally, A., Ernst, E., Lewith, G., MacFarlane, G. J. "Evidence for the efficacy of complementary and alternative medicines in the management of fibromyalgia: a systematic review." *Rheumatology*, March 2010. [Epub ahead of print].

Diatchenko, L., Slade, G. D., Nackley, A. G., Bhalang, K., Sigurdsson, A., et al. "Genetic basis for individual variations in pain perception and the development of a chronic pain condition." *Human Molecular Genetics*, 2005, 14(1): 135–143.

Fenollosa, P. "Rehabilitación. En España un 11% de personas padece diariamente dolor crónico". *Diario Médico*, December 31, 2010: 12.

Flor, H., Fydrich, T., Turk, D. C. "Efficacy of multidisciplinary pain treatment centres: a meta-analytic review." *Pain*, 1992, 49: 221–230.

Hoffman, B., Papas, R. K., Chatkoff, D. K., Kerns, R. D. "Meta-analysis of psychological interventions for chronic low back pain." *Health Psychology*, 2007, 26: 1–9.

Latremoliere, A., Woolf, C. J. "Central Sensitization: A Generator of Pain Hypersensitivity by Central Neural Plasticity." *The Journal of Pain*, 2009, 10(9): 895–926.

Leibing, E., Pfingsten, M., Bartman, U., et al. "Cognitive-behavioral treatment in unselected rheumatoid arthritis outpatients." *Clinical Journal of Pain*, 1999, 15: 58–66.

Manzanera, R. "Especial Dolor." *Diario Médico*, May 27, 2010: 17. [Interview]

Mayer, T., Polatin, P., Smith, B., et al. "Spine rehabilitation: secondary and tertiary nonoperative care." *The Spine Journal*, 2003, 3: 28S–36S.

McCracken, L. M., MacKichan, F., Eccleston, C. "Contextual cognitive-behavioral therapy for severely disabled chronic pain sufferers: Effectiveness and clinically significant chance." *European Journal of Pain*, 2007, 11: 314–322.

Miró Martínez, J. "Psicología del dolor." In *Tratamiento del Dolor. Teoría y Práctica*, 3rd ed. (Eds. L. Aliaga, J. E. Baños, C. Barutell, J. Molet, A. Rodríguez). Barcelona: Publicaciones Permanyer, 2009: 33–36.

Moix, J. "Análisis de los factores psicológicos moduladores del dolor crónico benigno." *Anuario de Psicologia*, 2005, 36: 37–60.

Moix, J. *Cara a cara con tu dolor. Técnicas y estrategias para reducir el dolor crónico*. Barcelona: Paidos, 2006.

Moix, J., Red Española de Investigadores en Dolencias de espalda. "Soporte psicológico al paciente con dolor crónico." Paper presentation at the III Forum Mediterráneo Multidisciplinar contra el Dolor. Menorca, Spain, May 9, 2009.

Mojaver, Y. N., Mosavi, F., Mazaherinezhad, A., Shahrdar, A., Manshaee, K. "Individualized homeopathic treatment of trigeminal neuralgia: an observational study." *Homeopathy*, 2007, 96(2): 82–86.

Nicholas, M. K., Wilson, P. H., Goyen, J. "Comparison of cognitive-behavioural group treatment and an alternative non-psychological treatment for chronic low back pain." *Pain*, 1992, 48: 339–347.

Nicholas, M. K. "When to refer to a pain clinic." *Best Practice & Research Clinical Rheumatology*, 2004, 18(4): 613–629.

Reichiling, D. B., Levine, J. D. "Critical role of nociceptor plasticity in chronic pain." *Trends in Neuroscience*, 2009, 32(12): 611–618.

Robinson, J. P., Allen, T., Fulton, L. D., Martin, D. "Perceived efficacy of pain clinics in the rehabilitation of injured workers." *Clinical Journal of Pain*, 1998, 14: 202–208.

Schonstein, E., Kenny, D., Keating, J., Koes, B., Herbert, R. D. "Physical conditioning programs for workers with back and neck pain: a cochrane systematic review." *Spine*, 2003, 28(19): E91–E95.

Shang, A., Huwiler-Müntener, K., Nartey, L., Juni, P., Dorig, S., Sterne, J. A., et al. "Are the clinical effects of homoeopathy placebo effects? Comparative study of placebo-controlled trials of homoeopathy and allopathy." *Lancet*, 2005, 366: 726–732.

Torres, et al. "El Ascensor Analgésico y la Escalera de la OMS." *Revista de la Sociedad Española del Dolor*, 2002, 9: 289–290.

Turner, J. A., Holtzman, S., Manel, Ll. "Mediators, moderators, and predictors of therapeutic change in congitive-behavioral therapy for chronic pain." *Pain*, 2007, 127: 276–286.

Turner, J. A., Manel, Ll., Aaron, L. A. "Short and long term efficacy of brief cognitive behavioral therapy for patients with chronic temporomandibular disorder pain: a randomized, controlled trial." *Pain*, 2006, 121: 181–194.

Vallejo Pareja, M. A. "Tratamiento psicológico del dolor crónico." *Boletín de Psicología*, 2005, 84(July).

Wasan, A. D., Gallagher, R. M. "Psychopharmacology for pain medicine." In *Essentials of Pain Medicine and Regional Anesthesia*, 2nd ed. (Eds. H. T. Benzon, S. N. Raja, R. E. Molloy, S. S. Liu, S. M. Fishman). Philadelphia: Churchill Livingstone, 2005: 124–133.

Wong, R., Wiffen, P. J. "Bisphosphonates for the relief of pain secondary to bone metastases." *Cochrane Database of Systematic Reviews*, 2002: CD002068.

World Health Organization. *Cancer pain relief: with guide to opioid availability*, 2nd ed. Geneva: World Health Organization, 1996.